Reasoning and Decision Making in Hematology

Reasoning and *Decision Making* in *Hematology*

Benjamin Djulbegović, M.D., Ph. D.
Assistant Professor
Division of Medical Oncology/Hematology
Department of Medicine
University of Louisville School of Medicine
Louisville, Kentucky

With contributions by

Sead Beganović, M.D., Ph. D.
Assistant Professor of Medicine
Department of Hematology
University Medical Center
Sarajevo, Bosnia and Herzegovina

Fred Hendler, M.D., Ph. D.
Associate Professor
Departments of Medicine and Biochemistry
University of Louisville School of Medicine
Louisville, Kentucky

Roger Herzig, M.D.
Marion F. Beard Professor
Department of Medicine
University of Louisville School of Medicine
Louisville, Kentucky

Geetha Joseph, M.D.
Assistant Professor
Department of Medicine
University of Louisville School of Medicine
Louisville, Kentucky

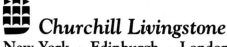

Churchill Livingstone
New York · Edinburgh · London · Melbourne · Tokyo

Library of Congress Cataloging-in-Publication Data

Djulbegović, Benjamin.
    Reasoning and decision making in hematology / Benjamin
Djulbegović, with contributions by Sead Beganović . . . [et al.].
        p. cm.
    Includes bibliographical references and indexes.
    ISBN 0-443-08858-6
    1. Hematology–Decision making. 2. Medical logic.   I. Beganović,
Sead. II. Title.
    [DNLM: 1. Decision Making. 2. Hematologic Diseases.   WH 100
D626r]
RC636.D55 1993
616.1'5–dc20
DNLM/DLC
for Library of Congress   92-49963
                                                           CIP

© **Churchill Livingstone Inc. 1992**

Distributed in the United Kingdom by Churchill Livingstone, Robert Stevenson House, 1–3 Baxter's Place, Leith Walk, Edinburgh EH1 3AF, and by associated companies, branches, and representatives throughout the world.

Accurate indications, adverse reactions, and dosage schedules for drugs are provided in this book, but it is possible that they may change. The reader is urged to review the package information data of the manufacturers of the medications mentioned.

The Publishers have made every effort to trace the copyright holders for borrowed material. If they have inadvertently overlooked any, they will be pleased to make the necessary arrangements at the first opportunity.

Acquisitions Editor: *Robert A. Hurley*
Copy Editor: *Barbara L. B. Storey*
Production Designer: *Jody L. Ouellette*
Production Supervisor: *Jeanine Furino*

Printed in the United States of America

First published in 1992   7 6 5 4 3 2 1

This book is dedicated to the people and the city of Sarajevo.

Life is short
And the art long
The occasion instant
Experiment perilous
Decision difficult
Hippocrates, c. 350 B.C.

Nature is probabilistic
And information incomplete
Outcomes are valued
Resources limited
Decision unavoidable
From Milton C. Weinstein and
Harvey V. Fineberg: Clinical Decision
Analysis, *WB Saunders, Philadelphia, 1980*

It has often been said that a person does not
really understand something until he teaches it
to someone else. Actually, a person does not
really understand something until he/she . . .
can express it as an algorithm.
D.E. Knuth, co-inventor of BASIC computer language

Preface

Reasoning and Decision Making in Hematology is intended for everyone who deals with the hematologic patient: students, residents, general internists, surgeons, and hematologists. It is the result of an attempt to apply decision theory and cognitive science concepts to hematologic problems. The book represents knowledge compiled from the current clinical practice of hematology. Original solutions to a variety of diagnostic and therapeutic problems are provided when adequate ones could not be compiled from the literature.

Our first goal is to identify the reasoning strategies that lie behind diagnostic and therapeutic problem solving in the care of patients with blood diseases. We have particularly tried to identify which kinds of hematologic problems are best approached with causal reasoning strategies, and which should be approached with probabilistic or deterministic (categorical) reasoning strategies. As a by-product of this approach, sets of *production rules* are identified in different areas of hematology. Where applicable, these rules, along with causal and/or probabilistic reasoning, are used to construct *algorithms* for teaching and for diagnostic/therapeutic problem solving in hematology. The text that accompanies each algorithm explains the principles behind its construction and also provides key clinical information. The reader is strongly encouraged to study these algorithms carefully. A problem-oriented (data-driven reasoning) method is applied in diagnostic situations. Whenever possible, we highlighted the preferred diagnostic approach. Here, the categorical and probabilistic approaches are mainly, but not exclusively, used. A disease-oriented (hypothesis-driven reasoning) approach is applied in the treatment settings. Here, causal and deterministic approaches and/or an estimate of the risk/benefit approach are mainly used.

Our second goal is to provide the clinician with guidelines and explicit details regarding two essential elements of clinical medicine: diagnostic and therapeutic decisions and actions. Such considerations include what test should be ordered; when should the test be ordered; what are the information values of our diagnostic armamentarium; what is the treatment of choice for a particular disorder; what are the optimal doses of drugs; how long should one administer a particular therapy; how is that therapy monitored; what is the optimal timing of certain therapeutic procedures; what is the time framework of clinical follow-up; and what is the most cost-effective strategy. Explicit guidelines (even when dealing with probabilistic estimates) are provided as they would be dictated by actual clinical practice. The reader not familiar with the basics of decision therapy and cognitive science concepts is advised to study the chapter "Decision Making, Algorithms, and Clinical Reasoning" before embarking on a specific hematologic topic. Quick information about the value of our diagnostic tools in hematology can be found with the help of the test sensitivity and specificity index.

Information is presented in a condensed algorithmic form, each algorithm summarizing tens of pages of written text. Here, we have sacrificed simplicity for thoroughness. We believe that the algorithms provide a core of hematologic information that, if presented discursively, would probably result in a textbook of a couple thousand pages in length. The lists of suggested readings that follow each chapter have been carefully selected to provide the reader with the most relevant and updated information. We believe that this book will be particularly useful not only to the busy clinician who needs quick solutions to hematologic problems but also for educational purposes, since it highlights the core of hematologic information.

No human endeavor, including writing a book, is an isolated experience. We want to thank all those who directly or indirectly helped in the creation of this work. In particular, we want to thank all our colleagues and staff at the Division of Hematology/Oncology of our Universities, without whose understanding and support this project would not have been possible. Special thanks go to Dr. Thomas Woodcock, Dr. Terence Hadley, and Dr. Richard Redinger, whose encouragement and help made this accomplishment possible. We are greatly indebted to Professor D. Hoelzer of the University of Johann Wolfgang Goethe in Frankfurt, Germany for providing us with the latest protocols for the treatment of adult acute lymphoblastic leukemia. We further thank Mr. Robert Hurley of Churchill Livingstone for sharing our enthusiasm and providing additional support toward the completion of this project. Also, many thanks go to Ms. Donna Vaughn, and at Churchill Livingstone, Ms. Barbara Storey and Ms. Donna Balopole, who did a marvelous job of editing the text, as well as to Ms. Melanie Hamilton, who helped us with the typing of the most complicated parts of the manuscript.

Last, but not least, we would be grateful for any advice, comments, or criticism, so that any potential future edition of this text can live up to the expectations of its readers.

Benjamin Djulbegović, M.D., Ph. D.
Sead Beganović, M.D., Ph. D.
Fred Hendler, M.D., Ph. D.
Roger Herzig, M.D.
Geetha Joseph, M.D.

Contents

III. WHITE BLOOD CELL PROBLEMS

High Count

Low Count

IV. ENLARGED LYMPH NODES/SPLEEN OR BONE PAIN

1 Decision Making, Algorithms, and Clinical Reasoning

An essential element of clinical practice is diagnostic and therapeutic problem solving. How this problem solving is accomplished is, however, not completely clear. To date, no theory of human problem solving has been accepted and no unified theory of clinical reasoning has been established. Studies on the cognitive aspects of clinical judgment have indicated that diagnosis is an *inferential* process, during which the clinician generates an hypothesis (*diagnostic triggering*). Hypotheses are continually being excluded or confirmed as new data are gathered. It has been estimated that a first hypothesis is generated 28 seconds after hearing the patient's chief complaint. An average of 5.5 hypotheses are generated for each case, and no more than seven hypotheses are active at any one time. The hypothesis forms a context (*model*) within which further information gathering takes place. *Verifying* a diagnostic hypothesis is the next step in the diagnostic process. Competing hypotheses are eliminated and an hypothesis that will serve as the basis for a patient's management is formed. Figure 1-1 shows the basic elements of this *hypothetico-deductive method.*

The essence of clinical medicine is the making of *decisions.* These decisions are made within a framework of imperfect information; we are never 100% sure when we make a diagnosis or start a new treatment. The clinical process, therefore, is highly probabilistic. Ideally, we would like to know the probabilities of all existing diagnostic possibilities, or estimates of so-called *pretest disease probability.* Hence, the importance of statistical data on the prevalence and incidence of disease. The role of new information, as gathered by ordering diagnostic tests,

is to increase the level of (diagnostic) certainty. However, our clinical tools are not perfect. It is of utmost importance that we understand the limitations of our tools; specifically, that we are able to *measure* the information they provide as precisely as possible. This is done by determining the *diagnostic test operating characteristics* (i.e., a set of characteristics that reflect information about patients with *and* without disease). These operating test characteristics are: *sensitivity, specificity, false-positive (α-error) and false-negative rate (β-error)* (see box for definitions of terms). Information content of diagnostic tests is best represented in terms of (Receiver Operating Characteristics) ROC plots. The ROC curve is a plot of sensitivity versus false-positive rate (Fig. 1-3A). When test characteristics are mathematically manipulated in conjunction with the pretest estimate of disease existence (Bayes' theorem), *post-test probability* of disease—the true estimate of the certainty level—can be calculated (Fig. 1-2 and box for formula). It is important, however, to realize that post-test probability *strongly* depends on the pretest probability (Fig. 1-3B and box for formulas). This will determine the actual usage of our diagnostic test armamentarium: the use of highly *sensitive* tests when we want to *exclude* disease and highly *specific* tests when we want to *confirm* diagnostic possibility (Fig. 1-4).

This probabilistic approach is very helpful in *hypothesis triggering.* However, care should be exercised with this approach; data on prevalence of disease and operating characteristics of diagnostic tests are not known in many instances. Bayes' theorem assumes that conditions are independent of each

Glossary of Terms and Useful "Decision Formulas"

Receiver operating characteristics (ROC): a set of characteristics that reflect the information a diagnostic test conveys about a patient with and without disease (sensitivity, specificity, false-negative, false positive rate)

Sensitivity (S) (true positives, TP): probability that a test will be positive when disease is present, $p(T+|D+)$

Specificity (Sp) (true negatives, TN): probability that a test result will be negative when disease is not present; $p(T-|D-)$

False-negative rate (FN = 1 − S): probability that a test result will be negative when disease is present; $p(T-|D+)$

False-positive rate (FP = 1 − Sp): probability that a test result will be positive when disease is not present; $p(T+|D-)$

Pretest probability [p(D+)]: probability that a condition exists before a test is performed (often means prevalence of a specific disorder, but can be related to the clinician's estimate of probability of disease before a test is performed)

Post-test probability of disease: probability of disease, given positive or a negative test result, $p(D+|T+)$ or $p(D+|T-)$

Bayes' theorem for calculating the post-test probability of disease:

$$p(D+|T+) = \frac{p(D+)*S}{p(D+)*S+(1-p(D+)*FP}$$

$$p(D+|T-) = \frac{p(D+)*FN}{p(D+)*FN+(1-p(D+)*Sp}$$

Formulas for calculation of decision thresholds:[a]

$$\text{Test-threshold} = \frac{FP*(\text{risk of inappropriate treatment}) + (\text{risk of diagnostic test})}{FP*(\text{risk of inappropriate treatment}) + S*(\text{benefit of treatment})}$$

$$\text{Treatment-threshold} = \frac{Sp*(\text{Risk of inappropriate treatment}) - (\text{risk of diagnostic test})}{Sp*(\text{risk of inappropriate treatment}) + FN*(\text{benefit of treatment})}$$

[a] Data from Pauker SG, Kassirer JP: The threshold approach to clinical decision making: N Engl J Med 302:1109, 1980

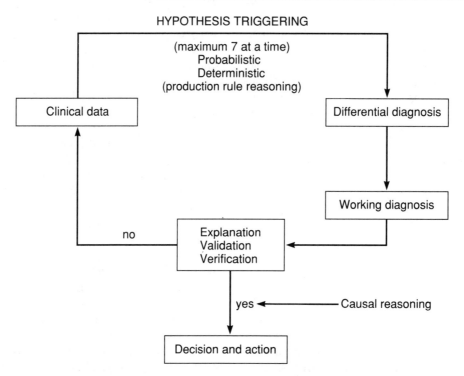

HYPOTHESIS TRIGGERING

Fig. 1-1. Hypothetico-deductive method of the diagnostic process. It can be argued that diagnosis is only a special case of the scientific method. In general, application of the probabilistic and production-rule reasoning is effective in hypothesis triggering, while causal reasoning is powerful in validating and verifying hypotheses.

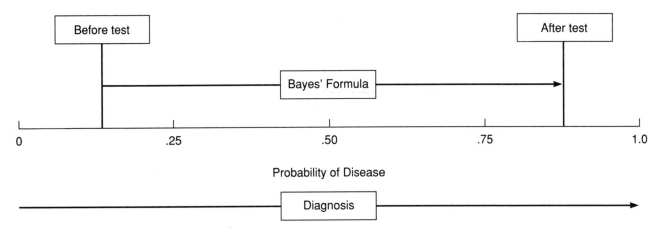

Fig. 1-2. The role of Bayes' theorem. Note how diagnostic certainty is increased after application of diagnostic test. (For Bayes' formula, see box, p. 2)—(From Sox et al.: Medical Decision Making. Butterworths, Boston, 1988, with permission.)

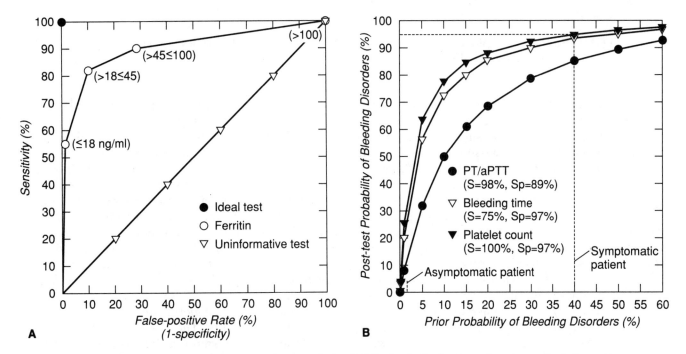

Fig. 1-3. **(A)** The receiver operating characteristics (ROC) plot is the best way to express the information content of diagnostic tests. The ROC curve is a plot of sensitivity *vs* false positive rate, each point on the curve being associated with a different threshold-decision level. The area under the curve of an ideal test is equal to 1 (S = 1, Sp = 1). ROC for a completely uninformative test corresponds to a 45° line. The performance of most tests is in between these two extremes. Note the inverse relationship between sensitivity and specificity—as one increases, the other decreases. (Data for ferritin ROC curve taken from Guayatt et al.: Diagnosis of iron-deficiency in elderly. Am J Med 88:205, 1990.) **(B)** Relation between pretest and post-test probability for positive test result. Note that the probability that disease actually exists in our patient strongly depends on the pretest probability of disease (prevalence, prior probability). Unexpected positive results in a patient with a low chance of having a specific disease should prompt us to re-evaluate its result. (For example, prolonged aPTT in an otherwise healthy forty-year-old male will result in only .12% that this patient actually has a clotting disorder; see Chapter 40.) Post-test probability if test is negative is a mirror picture of the above figure (see box, p. 2 for formulas with which these post-test probabilities can be calculated).

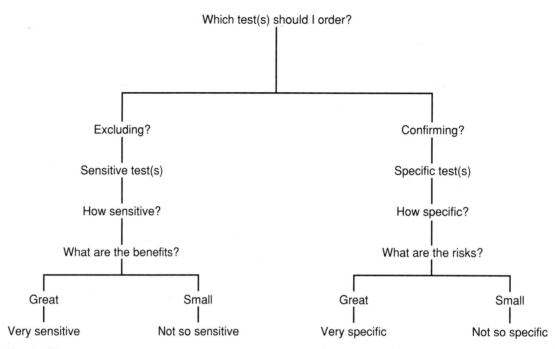

Fig. 1-4. Strategy for choice of diagnostic tests. (From Burke: Test strategies in selected clinical problems. Clin Labor Med 2:789, 1982, with permission.)

other, but this is often not true and may lead to miscalculation of our diagnostic certainty. Furthermore, the list of diagnostic possibilities must be exhaustive. If one diagnostic possibility is left out, it can never be taken into consideration as a possible explanation of a patient's symptoms.

Other reasoning strategies may therefore be helpful. Commonly used *heuristics* (mental processes used to learn, recall, or understand knowledge) are valuable rules of thumb that are an important aspect of clinical reasoning, particularly in hypothesis triggering. Two heuristics often used are the *availability heuristic* (diagnostic event is invoked because of the ease with which it is remembered); and the *representative heuristic* (diagnostic event is invoked because of the resemblance of a set of findings to a well-defined clinical entity). These heuristics are especially used in hematology because of the wide-spread use of routine hematological data such as a complete blood count (CBC), whose pattern of changes can trigger a diagnostic hypothesis after only a brief encounter with a patient.

When the pathophysiology of the process is known, the application of *causal reasoning* (cause-and-effect relationship) is a powerful method. While hypothesis triggering is not as successful with causal reasoning as with the probabilistic type, once an hypothesis is generated, the causal model is powerful in validating and verifying its strength (Fig. 1-1). Where ap-

plicable, causal reasoning remains an irreplaceable aspect of clinical reasoning.

Once a decision is made it is followed by action. Action is taken when the probability of disease exceeds a certain *decision threshold level*. In other words, at one particular moment in the diagnostic encounter, the physician has to decide whether disease exists or not, whether to order a test or not, and whether to treat a patient or not. At which level of diagnostic certainty a decision threshold will be reached depends on the operating characteristics of the test, the risk of the test, and the efficacy and risk of the treatment. Thus, diagnostic and treatment actions depend on the benefits and risks of diagnostic tests and treatments. The lower the ratio between benefit and risk, the more certain a diagnosis should be before giving the treatment (high *treatment threshold*), and vice versa. Generally, one may say that when benefits equal costs, the treatment threshold probability is equal to 0.50 (Fig. 1-5A). When disease probability is lower than the treatment threshold, the physician may order a diagnostic test to reduce *diagnostic entropy*, or do nothing. The probability at which these two choices have an equivalent value is called the *test threshold* (Fig. 1-5B and see box above for formulas on how to calculate threshold levels). A nomogram has been derived to enable easy determination of these thresholds, combining ROC characteristics of diagnostic

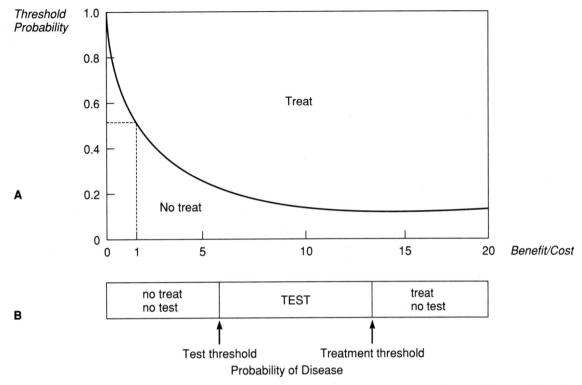

Fig. 1-5. **(A)** Threshold probability curve: relation between treatment threshold probability and benefit and cost (risk) of a treatment. Note that when benefit exceeds cost, the probability of disease at which we can start treatment is less than 50%.**(B)** Threshold concepts of decision making. Note the two thresholds: (1) test threshold probability, at which the choice between testing or not testing is equal and (2) treatment threshold probability, at which the choice between treating or not treating is equal. Action (to test or to treat) is taken when the probability of disease exceeds these decision threshold levels. Threshold probabilities are functions of operating characteristics of the test, risk of the test, and efficacy and risk of the treatment. These thresholds can be calculated according to the formula depicted in box on p. 2. (Fig. A from Pauker, Kassirer: A threshold approach to therapeutic decision making: a cost-benefit analysis. N Engl J Med 293:229, 1975, with permission.)

tests in the form of likelihood ratios (LR) and estimates of risk/benefit ratios (Fig. 1-6). In more general terms, this means that our decisions and actions are influenced by *probability* and *utility*. Practically, this can be translated as follows: determine the most common diagnosis first; then, consider diagnoses for which effective treatment exists (i.e., conditions with high benefit/risk ratios— "a diagnosis you can't afford to miss").

Most decisions in medicine are, however, straightforward and based upon *deterministic* or *categorical reasoning*, which is based upon compiled knowledge in a certain medical field. Use of the *production rules* (if/then) and *algorithms* are typical examples of this approach. As will be amply illustrated in this book, they may have origins in probabilistic or causal association between clinical findings.

An algorithm is an ordered set of instructions that analyzes a problem in step-by-step fashion and

makes diagnosing easier, especially for the novice. Clinical studies have shown that nurses guided by clinical algorithms are at least as effective as physicians in the diagnosis of certain complaints. They seem to be a more effective teaching method than prose, and are particularly suitable to overcoming information overload. For example, Work and Kunin's book, *Detection and Management of Urinary Tract Infection*, was reduced from 300 pages (representing findings from more than 500 articles) to one page with three algorithms! This reduction in itself may become the main reason for using algorithms, if one keeps in mind that medical knowledge is increasing exponentially, doubling in content every 10 years. To keep up with the ten leading journals in internal medicine, the clinician must read 200 articles and 70 editorials per month! Today, there are more than 20,000 biomedical journals. Furthermore, medical students are expected to learn

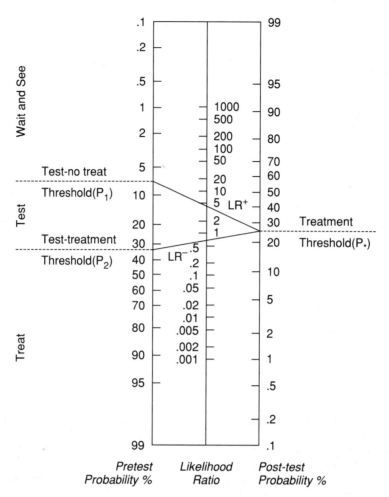

Fig. 1-6. Nomogram for determination of diagnostic and treatment threshold levels. To use the nomogram (1) decide on a treatment threshold, i.e., the probability above which you would treat and below which you would choose to wait; (2) mark this threshold on the post-test probability line of the nomogram; (3) rule backwards from the treatment threshold mark through the likelihood ratio of a positive test (LR+)—the intersection with pre-test probability is the test-no treat threshold; (4) rule backwards from the treatment threshold mark through the likelihood ratio of a negative test (LR−)—the intersection with pre-test probability is the test-treatment threshold. LR+ = sensitivity/false positive rate, LR− = false negative rate/specificity (From Glasziou: Threshold analysis via the Bayes' nomogram. Med Decis Making 11:61, 1991, with permission.)

130,300 bits of information, while a grand master chess player can recognize "only" 5,000 board patterns. It is estimated that a practicing physician needs more than 2 million bits of information for everyday work. Facing these facts, and acknowledging the brain's limited capacity for storage and processing of information, algorithms are becoming the best educational tool available.

There are problems with algorithms, however. They are usually unsuitable for patients with multiple problems because the standard starting point in the algorithm is identification of *one* particular problem (patient's complaints, abnormal diagnostic finding). They do not allow the clinician to bypass

essential steps in the clinical workup, and they usually become so complicated that it is difficult to present them as a ready-print figure. Nevertheless, we believe that the construction of algorithms based upon categorical and probabilistic reasoning represents the optimal way to teach hematology at the end of the twentieth century.

Suggested Readings

Holland RR: Decision tables: their use for the presentation of clinical algorithms. JAMA 233:455, 1975
Kassirer JP: Diagnostic reasoning. Ann Intern Med 110:893, 1989

Kassirer JP, Kopelman RI: Learning Clinical Reasoning. Williams & Wilkins, Baltimore, 1991

Moskowitz AJ, Kuipers BJ, Kassirer JP: Dealing with uncertainty, risks, and tradeoffs in clinical decisions: a cognitive science approach. Ann Intern Med 108:435, 1988

Sacket DL, Haynes RB, Guyatt GH, Tugwell P: Clinical Epidemiology. A Basic Science for Clinical Medicine. 2nd ed. Little, Brown, Boston, 1991

Sox HC, Blatt MA, Higgins M, Marton KI: Medical Decision Making. Butterworths, Boston, 1988

Szolovits P, Pauker SG: Categorical and probabilistic reasoning in medical diagnosis. Artificial Intelligence 11:115, 1978

2 | Approach to Hematologic Problems

Primary hematologic diseases are uncommon, while secondary hematologic problems occur rather frequently. A broad-based knowledge of medicine is therefore of utmost importance in dissecting hematologic disorders. The utility of the history and physical examination is limited in diagnosing primary hematologic disease, except when there is a strong positive family history for certain disorders (such as hemolytic disease or bleeding disorders), or when there are lymph nodes/spleen palpable on the physical exam, respectively. More information is often obtained from the laboratory tests. Hematologic disorders can be approached *anatomically* by identifying the compartment in the hematopoietic system that is affected: red blood cell, white blood cells, hemostasis, lymphopoietic system (Fig. 2-1). This is supplemented with a *physiologic* approach, which is based on the concept that biologic systems tend to self-regulate within narrow limits of some reference values. The major aberrations in the hematopoietic system are *quantitative* changes in the production of its particular constituent (excessive or deficient production). Primary *qualitative* abnormalities without quantitative changes are rarely observed in adults.* The reasoning strategy for arriving at a diagnosis of hematologic disorder is, then, to *combine* anatomic and physiologic assessment. Red blood cells are either low (anemia) or high (polycythemia). White blood cells are either high (leukocytosis) or low (leukopenia). Bleeding disorders

occur with increased or decreased platelets (thrombocytosis *vs* thrombocytopenia). Bleeding can occur due to a low concentration or biologic activity of important coagulation proteins, because of their low or abnormal production (hemophilia, von Willebrand's disease, etc.) or excessive destruction (DIC, fibrinolysis, etc.). The patient may have thrombosis due to a low concentration or low biologic activity of naturally occurring anticoagulants (antithrombin III, protein S deficiency, protein C deficiency, etc.) or increased platelets or red cells. Increased size of the lymph nodes and spleen can also be a reason for hematology consultation (Fig. 2-1).

On occasions, a patient will present with multiple hematologic problems. Although we have tried to highlight the "single hematologic problem" *vs* "multiple hematologic problems" approach in individual chapters (e.g., patient presenting with isolated anemia *vs* anemia as part of a three-lineage involvement), the challenge of proper identification of the hematologic problem will rest upon the reader of this text. In these cases, we advise consulting multiple chapters to arrive at a satisfactory solution to the problem.

The questions that a practitioner faces are: How abnormal must a diagnostic test be to indicate a diagnostic or therapeutic action? What are the *decision levels* of test(s), above or below which management action is recommended? What are those limiting values that can help us exclude or confirm certain diagnostic possibilities, or warn us that a significant physiologic effect is likely to occur?

It is important to notice that decision levels are not equal to abnormal results as defined by *normal*

---

* There are exceptions, however; e.g., bleeding occurring secondary to qualitative defects in the platelets.

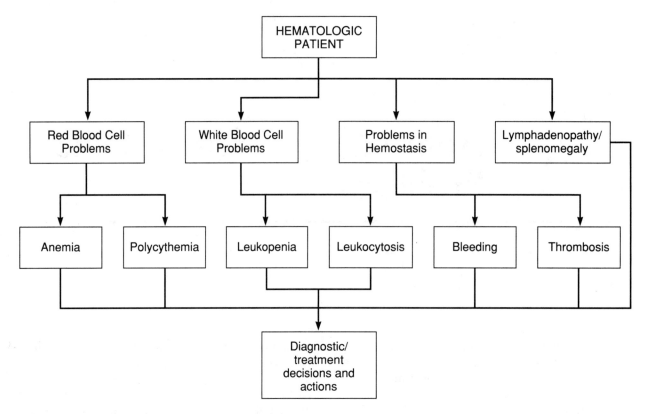

Fig. 2-1. An approach to hematologic problems. A combination of anatomic and physiologic approaches, as a variant to causal approaches (see Ch. 1), is the most useful general strategy. Threshold concept dominates further clinical workup.

interval or *reference range* for particular hematologic tests. Test results outside the reference range still do not mean that medical action will be taken (e.g., a platelet count of 120,000/mm³ in otherwise healthy pregnant women will require no action at all). Routine ordering of hematologic tests such as complete blood count (CBC) in an otherwise well patient (i.e., in low pretest probability setting) will result in approximately 5% abnormal result only (i.e., will be close to the expected deviation from the normal 95% reference range). This is the main reason why no hematologic test is indicated for screening purposes.

When benefits equal costs, the diagnostic probability at which treatment should be initiated is equal to 50% (see Chapter 1). If benefits and costs are not known, the majority of physicians would order a new diagnostic test at the level of diagnostic certainty of 25–30%. Therapy is usually administered when they are 65–70% confident of the diagnosis. For common hematologic tests, action will be taken if results change in reference values from 3.2–16.4% (Table 2-1).

Table 2-1. Coefficient of Variations (CV) of Decision Levels for Common Hematologic Diagnostic Tests[a]

Diagnostic Test	Decision Level	Medically Useful CV (%)
Hematocrit (%)	42	5.4
Hemoglobin (g/dl)	13–15 (130–150 g/L)	3.6
Leukocyte (mm³)	5,000	16.4
Leukocyte (mm³)	25,000	14
MCV (fl)	95	3.2
Prothrombin time (sec)	12.5–20	15.2

[a] (Modified from Skenzdel et al: Am J Clin Pathol 40:200, 1985, with permission)

Table 2-2. Decision Levels for Common Hematologic Tests[a]

Diagnostic Test	Decision Level	Comments
Antithrombin III	<50% normal level	Risk for spontaneous thrombosis
Bleeding time	>20 min	Risk for spontaneous bleeding
Fibrinogen	<30 mg/dl (<0.3 g/L)	Risk for spontaneous hemorrhage
Hematocrit	14%	Consider transfusion
	55% (female)	Always due to true increment in red blood cell mass
	60% (male)	Always due to true increment in red blood cell mass
	70%	Phlebotomy urgently indicated
Hemoglobin	<4.5 g/dl (>45 g/L)	Transfusion indicated
	<10.0 g/dl (<100.0 g/L)	Anemia workup indicated
	>17.0 g/dl (>170.0 g/L) (female)	High probability of true increment in red blood cell mass
	>18.0 g/dl (>180.0 g/L) (male)	High probability of true increment in red blood cell mass
	>23.0 g/dl (>230.0 g/L)	Urgent phlebotomy indicated
PTT	<1.5 × control	No bleeding risk
	>2.5–3 × control (>90 sec)	Risk for spontaneous bleeding
PT	<1.5 × control	No bleeding risk
	>2.5 × control	Risk for spontaneous bleeding
Platelet count	<5,000–10,000/mm^3 (5–10 × 10^9/L)	Risk for spontaneous bleeding
	10,000–50,000 (10–50 × 10^9/L)	Bleeding risk upon trauma
	>2,000,000 (>2,000 × 10^9/L)	Risk for thrombosis/bleeding
Vitamin B$_{12}$	<100 pg/ml (<7.4 pmol/L)	Strongly suggests pernicious anemia (vitamin B$_{12}$ therapy)
Leukocyte	<500/mm^3 (.5 × 10^9/L)	Great risk for infection
	>100,000 (blasts)/mm^3	Risk for leukostasis; urgent therapy indicated
	Blasts in the smear	Urgent workup indicated

[a] Levels are derived from the physiologic relationship between test and condition it measures; note that it only points to the increased *likelihood* that events will occur. How likely it is that event will occur can be calculated using Bayes' theorem and the "threshold" formulas (see boxed list in Chapter 1).

Precise decision levels can only be determined through a formal decision analysis, which considers the test operating characteristics for the disease in question, risk of the test, and efficacy and risk of the treatment (see Chapter 1). Where available, this data will be presented in individual chapters. When the results of decision analyses are not available, a physiologic (causal) approach (see Chapter 1) can be used to define levels when physiologic aberrations are expected to occur. Table 2-2 summarizes some of the decision levels related to common hematologic diagnostic tests.

Suggested Readings

Ruttiman S, Clemencon D, Dubach UC: Usefulness of complete blood counts as a case-finding tool in medical outpatients. Ann Intern Med 116:44, 1992

Shapiro MF, Greenfield S: The complete blood count and leukocyte differential count. Ann Intern Med 106:65, 1987

Skendzel LP, Barnett RN, Platt R: Medically useful criteria for performance of laboratory tests. Am J Clin Pathol 40:200, 1985

Statland BE: Clinical Decision Levels for Lab Tests. Medical Economics, Oradell, NJ, 1984

Williams WJ: Approach to the Patient. In Williams WJ, et al. (eds): Hematology. 4th Ed. McGraw-Hill, New York, 1990

Wintrobe MM: The Diagnostic and Therapeutic Approach to Hematologic Problems. In Wintrobe MM (ed): Clinical Hematology. 8th Ed. Lea & Febiger, Philadelphia, 1981

3 | Anemia: Diagnosis*

Anemia is the most common hematologic disorder; 20% of hospital admissions among the elderly are due to anemia. According to the World Health Organization (WHO) criteria, anemia is diagnosed in males if the hematocrit is less than 0.39 (39%) and the hemoglobin is less than 130 g/L (13 g/dl). In females, a hematocrit of less than 0.36 (36%) and a hemoglobin of less than 120 g/L (12 g/dl) is a diagnosis of anemia. An optimal diagnosis of anemia involves the combination of *probabilistic, morphologic* and *physiologic* approaches (Fig. 3-1). The latter two approaches are variants of the causal approach, as discussed in Chapter 1. These three reasoning strategies are by no means exclusive, and, in effect, are firmly interwoven in the clinical workup. The principle of availability heuristic is widely incorporated in the diagnostic strategy of anemia as well, partly because of the widespread use of electronic counters for determination of the complete blood count (CBC).

Traditionally, morphologic data is used to classify an anemic state. For decades physicians have relied upon the use of red blood cell (RBC) indices, examination of the peripheral smear, and physical examination of the patient.

How good are our tools for diagnosing anemia? Table 3-1 shows the values of our diagnostic armamentarium in the diagnosis of anemia. It should be noted that the absence of pallor or other *physical* signs of anemia does not rule out anemia (an average

false-negative value is about 45–55%). An examination of the peripheral smear performs no better than RBC indices alone. Overall, it provides unique diagnostic information in only 4–6% of cases and additional helpful information in the diagnosis of another 25% of blood disorder cases. RBC indices, also, are associated with too many false-positives and false-negatives to be of great practical use. Thus, a traditional approach is far from being infallible in the correct diagnosis of anemia.

A probabilistic approach can be effectively combined with the traditional approach. Figure 3-1 shows the prevalence of different types of anemias in the U.S. population. The diagnosis of specific anemic disorders, or positive test predictive values, will therefore depend on test operating characteristics and the prevalence of anemia (i.e., its pretest probability). It should be noted that by far the most common type of anemia is iron deficiency anemia (IDA), followed by thalassemia and anemia of chronic disease (ACD).

An effective diagnostic workup therefore starts with a question: Does this patient have iron deficiency anemia or another type of anemia? The construction of the anemia algorithm in Figure 3-2 is based on these principles. In the majority of cases, further workup will depend on whether IDA is excluded or not (Fig. 3-2). Here, the major problem lies in distinguishing between IDA and ACD (see Chapter 5). It is worth mentioning that 75% of all hospital anemias are caused by IDA or ACD.

The principle of decision analysis teaches that additional testing should be performed only if subsequent management will differ upon obtaining the

---

* See individual chapters for further discussion of diagnosis and treatment of specific types of anemia.

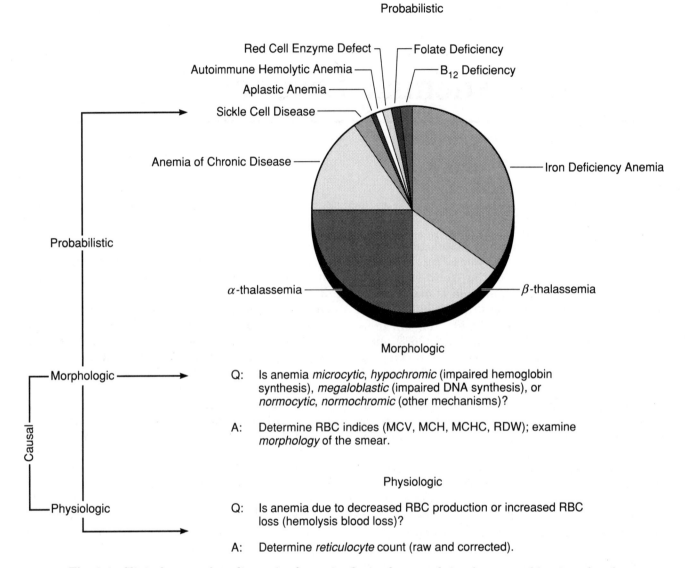

Probabilistic

Red Cell Enzyme Defect ⌐ ⌐Folate Deficiency
Autoimmune Hemolytic Anemia ─┐ ⌐B$_{12}$ Deficiency
Aplastic Anemia ─┐
Sickle Cell Disease ─┐

Anemia of Chronic Disease ─── ─── Iron Deficiency Anemia

α-thalassemia ─── ─── β-thalassemia

Probabilistic

Causal

Morphologic

Physiologic

Morphologic

Q: Is anemia *microcytic, hypochromic* (impaired hemoglobin synthesis), *megaloblastic* (impaired DNA synthesis), or *normocytic, normochromic* (other mechanisms)?

A: Determine RBC indices (MCV, MCH, MCHC, RDW); examine *morphology* of the smear.

Physiologic

Q: Is anemia due to decreased RBC production or increased RBC loss (hemolysis blood loss)?

A: Determine *reticulocyte* count (raw and corrected).

Fig. 3-1. Clinical approach to diagnosis of anemia. Optimal approach involves a combination of *probabilistic, morphologic,* and *physiologic* clinical reasoning (see also boxed material p. 17). The latter two approaches are variants of the causal approach (see Ch. 1). Note that "corrected" reticulocyte count provides evidence regarding RBC production (reticulocyte production index), and that "raw" reticulocyte count is an index of RBC life span.

Table 3-1.[a] Operating Characteristics of Common Tests Used in Diagnosis of Anemia

Test	Sensitivity (%)	Specificity (%)	Disease
Physical Exam			
Pallor	48–67	58–71	Anemia (hematocrit = 30%)
(face, conjunctivae, nailbeds, palms)			
Palmar creases	12	98	Anemia (hematocrit = 30%)
Splenomegaly	97–100	30–50 (?)	Hereditary spherocytosis
Lab Blood Smear Reading			
Microcytosis	16–63	53–95	Iron deficiency anemia
Macrocytosis	4–84	69–94	Vitamin B_{12} deficiency/FAD
Hypersegmented neutrophils (5 cells with 5 lobes or 1 cell with 6 lobes)	91–95	77	Vitamin B_{12} deficiency/FAD
RBC Indices			
RDW > 15	87–100	66	Iron deficiency anemia
MCV < 100	100	15–30	Iron deficiency anemia
MCV < 84	48	75	Iron deficiency anemia
MCV < 80	100	30–50(?)	Thalassemia
MCV > 105	11	95	Vitamin B_{12} deficiency/FAD
MCHC > 36	100 (?)	95–100	Hereditary spherocytosis
Common Lab Tests			
Ferritin < 12 ng/ml	65–97	99	Iron deficiency anemia
Transferrin saturation < 16%	95–100	70–95	Iron deficiency anemia
Reticulocyte count (%)	62–90	99[b]	Hemolysis
Coombs test	96–98	92–95	Autoimmune hemolytic anemia (all reagents)
Hemosiderin (urine)	100	?	PNH
Low vitamin B_{12} (<200)	90–95	95 (?)	B_{12} deficiency
Anti-intrinsic factor antibody	60–70	>99	Pernicious anemia
Achlorhydria	100	30–50 (?)	Pernicious anemia

[a] See individual chapters for more ROC data.

Abbreviations: FAD, folic acid deficiency; PNH, paroxysmal nocturnal hemoglobinuria; MCV, mean cell volume; MCHC, mean cell hemoglobin concentration; RDW, red (cell) distribution width.

[b] If >10%.

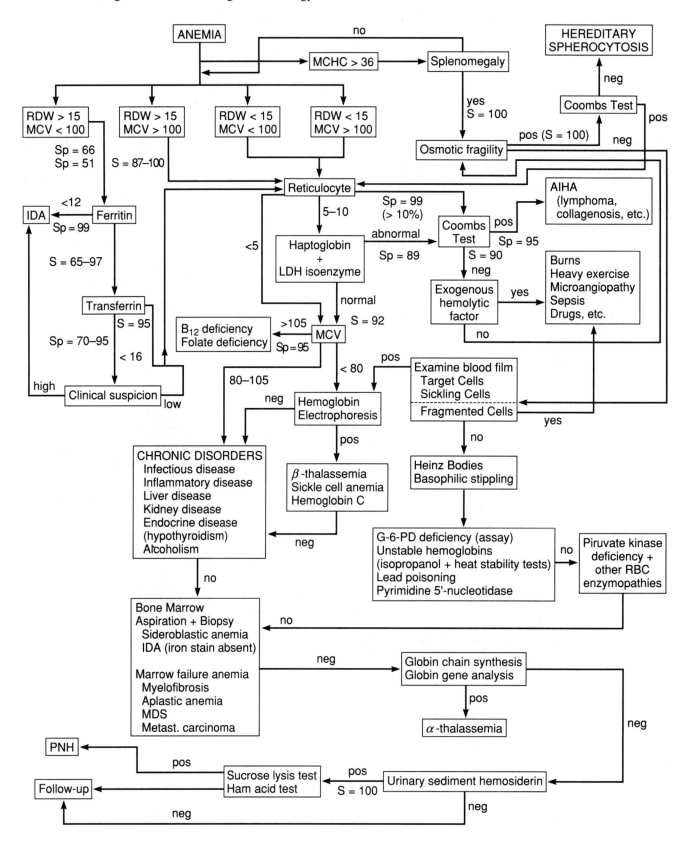

Production Rules When Anemia Presents Along With Involvement of Other Cell Lines

_____

1. *If* anemia is associated with leukopenia/thrombocytopenia, *then* think of primary marrow disease (PMD—e.g., AA, MPS, MDS, AL, MPh, PA, viral disease) or (1) hypersplenism or (2) Evans syndrome (rare condition), (3) MAHA (look for shistocytes in the peripheral smear)

2. *If* reticulocytes are *not* increased, *then* think of PMD and perform bone marrow aspiration/biopsy.

3. *If* reticulocytes are increased and MAHA (normal smear/non-specific smear) or hypersplenism (normal liver spleen/scan) or Evans syndrome are not diagnosed (Coombs test negative), *then* suspect paroxysmal nocturnal hemoglobinuria.

_____

Abbreviations: AA, aplastic anemia; MPS, myeloproliferative syndrome (late complications); MDS, myelodysplastic syndrome; AL, acute leukemia; MPh, myelophthisic anemia; PA, pernicious anemia; MAHA—microangiopathic hemolytic anemia. See also boxed material in Chapters 8 and 27, and Figure 40-3B.

---

new information. This is the reason why thalassemia, although a highly prevalent condition, need not be tested upfront; by and large, no therapy will be indicated (see Chapter 9).

When IDA is excluded, the physiologic approach, with its determination of reticulocyte counts, is the most powerful. It will answer the question of whether anemia is due to decreased RBC production or increased RBC blood destruction. Additional help in answering this question may come from the presence/absence of lymphadenopathy/splenomegaly and a combination of this piece of information with RBC indices (e.g., low reticulocyte and high mean cell volume (MCV) directs a workup for megaloblastic anemias). Further approaches may become probabilistic again (e.g., what is the most common hemolytic anemia, etc.).

If anemia is present along with the involvement of other cell lines, an optimal approach may involve application of the *production rule*, as presented in the boxed material below.

One should remember that anemia is not a disease but rather a *sign* of disease. Once a diagnosis is established, the physician should ask himself/herself: What caused this patient's (iron deficiency, megaloblastic, hemolytic, etc.) anemia?

Suggested Readings

Beutler E: Common anemias. JAMA 259:2433, 1988

Crosby WH: Reticulocyte counts. Arch Intern Med 141:1747, 1981

Djulbegovic B, Hadley T, Pasic R: A new algorithm for diagnosis of anemia. Postgrad Med 85:119, 1989

Jen P, Woo B, Rosenthal P, Bunn F, et al. The value of the peripheral smear in anemic inpatients. The laboratory's reading *v* a physician's reading. Arch Intern Med 143:1120, 1983

Nardonne DA, Roth KM, Mazur DJ, McAfee JH: Usefulness of physical examination in detecting the presence or absence of anemia. Arch Intern Med 150:201, 1990

Steinberg MH, Dreillng BJ: Microcytosis: its significance and evaluation. JAMA 249:85, 1983

Fig. 3-2. Algorithm for diagnosis of anemia. An algorithm is constructed upon principles outlined in Fig. 3-1 and the availability of data, which will trigger a certain diagnostic hypothesis (availability heuristic). If the anemia is part of a three-lineage involvement, apply the production rule in boxed material above. (MCV, mean red cell volume; RDW, red cell distribution width; MCHC, mean red cell hemoglobin concentration; AIHA, autoimmune hemolytic anemia; PNH, paroxysmal hemolytic anemia; IDA, iron deficiency anemia; MDS, myelodysplastic syndrome) (See boxed material in Chapters 6 and 8, and Figs. 9-1 and 12-1 for a more detailed approach to diagnosis of specific classes of anemia; see also individual chapters for further diagnostic and therapeutic considerations.) (From Djulbegovic et al.: Postgrad Med 85:119, 1989, with permission.)

4 | Anemia: Treatment*

When to treat anemia? In order to answer this question, one must ask whether the anemia itself contributes to significant morbidity and mortality. It seems that profound, symptomatic anemia *does* significantly contribute to the patient's morbidity and mortality. The mortality rate in patients with a hemoglobin as low as 3 g/dl (30 g/L) is as high as 87%. On the other hand, it seems that no morbid effects from mild anemia exist when it is not associated with an underlying disease; patients with anemia due to chronic failure may tolerate a hemoglobin level of less than 7 g/dl (70 g/L). Compensatory increases in cardiac output can readily maintain adequate tissue oxygenation at hematocrit levels as low as 20–25%. No difference in the mortality rate between normal persons and those with mild anemia was found when death due to malignancies were excluded. Thus, threshold levels for the treatment of anemia can be derived from these expected physiologic consequences of low hemoglobin on tissue oxygenation. This is a causal model of clinical reasoning.

Treatment decision levels. While these levels may vary in individual patients, for initiation of therapy one may apply (as a general rule) the following decision levels:

Hematocrit 30–36% and hemoglobin 8.0–12.0 g/dl (80–120 g/L)

Generally, no action is indicated. Comfortable physical activity is usually achieved at hemoglobin levels between 7.0–8.0 g/dl (70–80 g/L) with a normal cardiovascular system, or with a hemoglobin >9.0 g/dl (>90 g/L) in the presence of coronary heart disease.

Hematocrit 14–30% and hemoglobin 4.5–8.0 g/dl (45–80 g/L)

Further action depends on the clinical setting. Usually, diagnostic evaluation would be indicated prior to instituting therapy.

Hematocrit ≤14% and hemoglobin ≤4.5 g/dl (≤45 g/L)

Therapeutic intervention is indicated. One has to be aware of the clinical settings of this intervention (e.g., cautious approach in the speed of delivery of transfusion in cardiac heart failure, aggravation of pain due to anemia hypoxia in coronary heart disease, etc.).

How to treat anemia? Treatment is directed toward a specific cause of the anemia (see individual chapters). In general, a transfusion is indicated in the setting of profound, symptomatic anemia. This decision will be guided by the principles of risk *vs* benefit of the transfusion in individual patients (see Chapters 50, 51).

---

* See individual chapters for specific treatments.

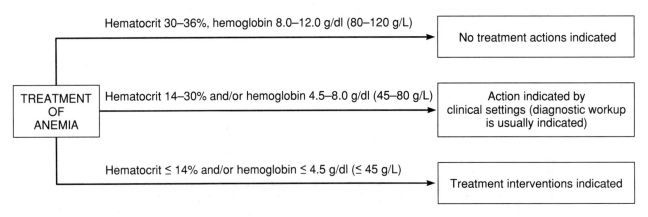

Fig. 4-1. Anemia treatment threshold levels. These levels are derived from the expected physiologic consequences of the low hemoglobin level on tissue oxygenation (causal model of clinical reasoning). (Note that these guidelines apply to normovolemic or hypervolemic patients. Hypovolemia further decreases tissue oxygen delivery, regardless of hemoglobin level.)

Suggested Readings

Elwood DC, Waters WE, Benjamin IT, Sweetnam PM: Mortality and anemia in women. Lancet i:891, 1974

Shapiro MF, Greenfield S: The complete blood count and leukocyte differential count. An approach to their rational application. Ann Intern Med 106:65, 1987

Statland BE: Clinical Decision Levels for Laboratory Tests. Medical Economics Books, Oradell, NJ, 1984

Zauder HL: Preoperative hemoglobin requirements. Anesthesiol Clin North Am 8:471, 1990

5 | Iron Deficiency Anemia

Iron deficiency anemia (IDA) is one of the most common disorders of mankind, and doubtless the most common hematologic disease. It affects about 30% of the world's population. In the U.S. it affects between 0.2–2% of the adult male population and between 2–10% of the adult female population. It is commonly undiagnosed because its clinical symptoms are subtle, with the major effect being upon productivity and work performance. The likelihood of IDA development increases to about 60% in pregnant women, 80% in heavily menstruating women, and more than 90% in those individuals with pica symptoms. (A heavy menstrual blood loss is usually defined as > 300 ml/period or > 10 tampons/pads per period; note that as little as 5 ml of blood loss containing 2.5 mg of iron matches the ability of the intestine to absorb iron.) These figures can be used as relating to the pretest probabilities of IDA. Diagnosing IDA is, in fact, relatively simple. Although the gold standard for diagnosis is the demonstration of iron stores in bone marrow, in the majority of cases this test would not be necessary. Diagnosis of IDA can be effectively ruled out by normal red (cell) distribution width (RDW) or transferrin (RDW sensitivity = 87–100%, transferrin sensitivity = 95–99%). Low ferritin confirms a diagnosis of IDA (specificity = 99–100%) (Table 5-1).

Clinical problems arise in distinguishing between IDA and *anemia of chronic disease* (ACD), in that both present with low serum iron (Table 5-2). A highly specific test, such as ferritin, is of no help here because it is an acute phase-reactant, and the patient may have falsely high ferritin and complicating IDA. Such typical scenarios can be seen in pa-

tients with rheumatoid arthritis who are taking aspirin or other nonsteroidal antirheumatic agents where risk from gastrointestinal bleeding is a real threat. In such cases, corrections of the ferritin level for underlying inflammatory processes, based upon the erythrocyte sedimentation rate or other laboratory parameters, may be quite useful (Fig. 5-1). It is worthwhile to repeat that 75% of all hospital anemias are caused by IDA or ACD. Frequently, the question of a patient having IDA will be raised because of the microcytosis routinely found on the complete blood count (CBC). As can be seen from Table 5-1, the specificity of mean cell volume (MCV) is very low and cannot be used to diagnose IDA. Figure 9-1 shows the approach to microcytic anemia.

While replacement therapy with iron (Fig. 5-2) is the logical procedure, an *etiologic* approach is essential in the treatment of IDA. One should always ask *why* this patient has IDA. The major causes of IDA come from *blood loss* (menstruation, gastrointestinal bleeding, bleeding from the urinary tract, etc.), *decreased absorption* (gastric surgery, dietary insufficiency, malabsorption, etc.; one has to remember that, except following a gastrectomy, isolated malabsorption of iron is extremely rare), or *increased requirement* (pregnancy, infants, etc.; supplementary iron and folic acid is indicated from the fourth month of pregnancy). Figure 5-3 shows the threshold approach to diagnostic and treatment strategies in IDA in the function of the given ferritin value. Depending on the estimate of *benefit/cost ratio*, testing and treatment threshold levels vary considerably for the same ferritin value. This means that iron replacement therapy can be started in women of child-

Table 5-1. Operating Test Characteristics of Common Tests in Diagnosis of Iron Deficiency Anemia

Diagnostic Test	Sensitivity (%)	Specificity (%)
Iron (<50 µg/ml)	100	54
Iron (<17 µg/ml)	57	90
MCV (mean red blood cell volume) (<100 fl)	100	15–30
MCV (<80 fl)	27	75–91
Red (cell) distribution width (>15%)	87–100	66
Percent of saturation of transferrin (<16%)	95–99	70–95
Percent of saturation of transferrin (<8%)	61	85
Serum ferritin (<12 ng/ml)	65–97	99–100
Ferritin (<45 ng/ml)	82	90
RBC protoporphyrin (>2)	47	84

(Red cell ferritin may be more sensitive and specific than serum ferritin.)

Table 5-2. Common Diagnostic Problem: Distinction Between Iron Deficiency Anemia (IDA) and Anemia of Chronic Disease (ACD)[a]

	Normal Range	IDA (mean)	ACD (mean)
Iron (µg/ml)	70–90	30	30
Iron-binding capacity	250–400	450	200
Percent of saturation	30	7	15
Marrow iron	2+	0	3+
Ferritin (ng/ml)	20–220	10	150
RBC ferritin	4–28	3.5	9.7

[a] Data from Erslev: Anemia of chronic disease. In Williams WJ et al. (eds): Hematology 4th Ed. McGraw-Hill, New York, 540, 1990 and Balaban EP et al.: Blood 72:37a, 1988

months following correction of the anemia, to replete iron stores. If a response is not noted, one should suspect the accuracy of the diagnosis; the most common mistake is treating patients who have an anemia of chronic disorder or thalassemia with iron.

The response rate to oral iron is not lower than

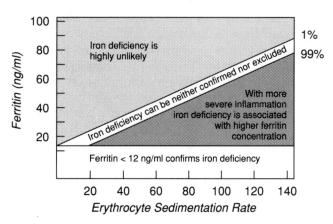

Fig. 5-1. Estimation of the probability of iron deficiency anemia in patients with underlying inflammatory disease. The graph shows the estimated correction of the ferritin level as an acute phase reactant for the level of an erythrocyte sedimentation rate. The graph is shown to illustrate a concept, and may not be applicable to individual patients. Another approach is to use a *production rule*: suspicion of IDA in the presence of conditions known to cause ACD if ferritin < 60 ng/ml (or <110 ng/ml in patients with rheumatoid arthritis). (From Witte et al.: Am J Clin Pathol 85:202, 1986, with permission.)

bearing age with a probability of disease as low as 7%, but would not begin before a certainty of diagnosis higher than 90% in adult males. This difference in the benefit/cost ratio estimate is the consequence of the probability of the etiology of IDA in childbearing women and adult males, with menorrhagia being the most common in the former and gastrointestinal bleeding in the latter group. For this reason, every adult male suspected of IDA should be tested for occult blood in the stool as part of the routine clinical workup.

The ultimate proof of a diagnosis of IDA is response to treatment; anemia should be corrected within 2 months, with an approximate build-up rate of hemoglobin of 2 g/L/day. The optimal dosage is about 65 mg of elemental iron (200 mg of ferrous sulfate exsiccated) three times a day between meals. Plain ferrous sulfate is still the best choice for treatment, which should be continued for at least 6–8

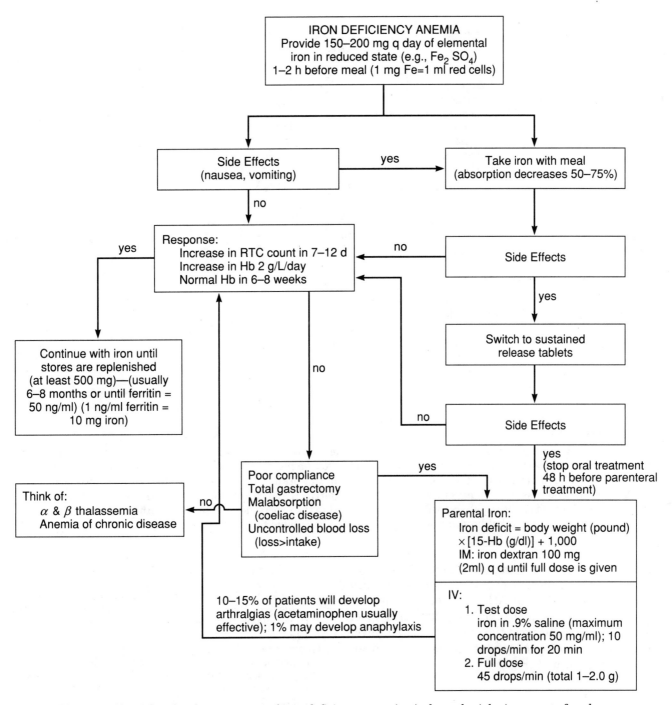

Fig. 5-2. Algorithm for the treatment of iron deficiency anemia. A clear *physiologic concept* of replacement treatment determines all practical aspects of the therapy of iron deficiency anemia.

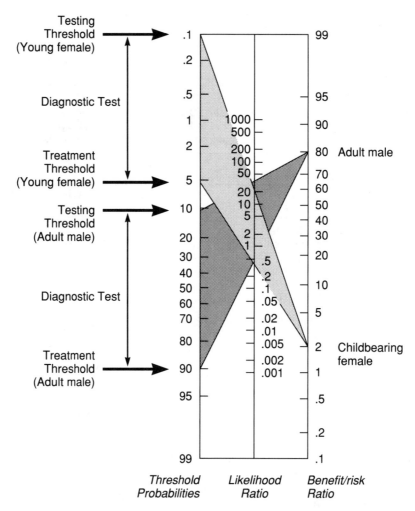

Fig. 5-3. Threshold approach to iron deficiency anemia (IDA). Critical decisions in IDA include when further exploration of etiologic explanations of IDA (*diagnostic threshold*) is indicated and when to undertake immediate treatment without further clinical workup (*treatment threshold*). These thresholds will depend upon the results of the particular test (ferritin) and the estimated risk/benefit ratio, where the expected benefit to patients with disease is equal to the expected "cost" to those without disease (see also Chapter 1). (Likelihood ratios for ferritin levels calculated for the level < 20 ng/ml.)

the rate of response to parenteral treatment. Thus, parenteral iron therapy should be avoided as a routine way of treating IDA because of possible side-effects, such as anaphylactic shock, urticaria, fever, and pain and swelling at the injection site. However, in a certain number of patients, parenteral iron still might be indicated (Fig. 5-3).

Suggested Readings

Beck JR: The role of new laboratory test in clinical decision making. Clin Lab Med 2:751, 1982

Cook JD, Skikne BS: Iron deficiency: definition and diagnosis. J Intern Med 226:349, 1989

Fairbanks VF, Beutler E: Iron deficiency anemia. In Williams WJ, Beutler E, Erslev AJ, Licthman MA (eds): Hematology, 4th Ed. McGraw-Hill, New York, 482, 1990

Guayatt G, Patterson C, Ali M, et al.: Diagnosis of iron deficiency anemia in the elderly. Am J Med 88:205, 1990

Pasquala D, Divakara M, Tsan MF, et al.: The utility of noninvasive tests for assessment of iron stores. Blood 76:44a, 1990

Scrimshaw NS: Iron deficiency. Sci Am October:46, 1991

Witte DL, Kraemer DF, Johnson GF, et al.: Prediction of bone marrow findings from tests performed on peripheral blood. Am J Clin Pathol 85:202, 1986

6 | Megaloblastic Anemia

Ninety-five percent of cases of *megaloblastic anemia* are caused by vitamin B_{12} and folate acid deficiency, respectively. These deficiencies occur at the level of *decreased intake, impaired absorption,* or *increased requirement* (see box below). The human body has a reserve of about 3–6 months of folate acid

---

Pathophysiologic Approach to Etiology of Megaloblastic Anemia

Decreased Intake
Folate Acid
    Alcoholism, poor nutrition, old age
    Hemodialysis, hyperalimentation
    Goat's milk anemia, premature infants
Vitamin B_{12}
    Vegetarianism

Impaired Absorption
Folate Acid
    Nontropical sprue
    Tropical sprue
    Small intestinum diseases
Vitamin B_{12}
    Pernicious anemia
    Gastrectomy
    Zollinger-Ellison syndrome
    Ileal resection or Crohn's disease
    Fish tapeworm
    Blind loop syndrome
    Pancreatic insufficiency

Increased Requirements
Folate Acid
    Pregnancy
    Hemolytic anemia
    Exfoliative dermatitis

---

and 3–5 years of vitamin B_{12}, and deficiencies are expected to develop after this period of time. Abnormalities at the level of the gastrointestinal tract are almost always underlying pathogenic mechanisms responsible for vitamin B_{12} and folate deficiencies. The most common cause of folate deficiency is malnutrition (i.e., inadequate dietary intake), which is nearly universal among chronic alcoholic patients. Malabsorption, on the other hand, is almost always the mechanism responsible for vitamin B_{12} deficiency, of which pernicious anemia (PA) is the most common cause. As many as 7% of the elderly population can be expected to have a vitamin B_{12} deficiency. The annual incidence of PA is estimated to be about 100 per million population. The disease is usually present around the age of 60, commonly affecting persons of Scandinavian origin (about .13% of the population). While it attacks only 2–6% of the white population younger than 40 years, it can affect up to 21% of black individuals below the age of 40. A *causal* approach to these conditions would ideally require full documentation of the deficiency state, an estimate that the deficiency is responsible for anemia or other clinical conditions, and, finally, identification of the pathologic condition that is causing the deficiency. However, this is not only frequently impossible, but also does not seem desirable (see below).

The principle of availability heuristic is incorporated in the traditional approach to megaloblastic anemia. The clinician would suspect megaloblastic anemia after an increased mean cell volume (MCV) in the routine complete blood count (CBC) is found. There are other causes of increased MCV, however (see box below), and most importantly, *a normal MCV does not exclude megaloblastic anemia*. Because tests that help us in documenting vitamin B_{12}/folate deficiencies are far from being perfect (Table 6-1 and box below), a diagnosis will generally be highly probabilistic. Furthermore, since benefit/risk ratio for the treatment of these conditions is so high, a case can be made that a patient with a low probability of B_{12}/folate deficiencies should be treated without aggressively pursuing the diagnosis (Fig. 6-1). This would particularly apply to patients with vitamin B_{12} deficiency who may experience neuropsychiatric disorders in the absence of any hematologic abnormalities. Since the payoff is so high, and the risk of the treatment is so low, it is now recommended that *any* patient with suspected vitamin B_{12} deficiency be given a *therapeutic trial of 4 months of treatment*.

In general, one should avoid transfusions in the treatment of megaloblastic anemia, especially in PA patients, because of the danger of acute pulmonary edema in patients with chronic anemia. Also, the dose of vitamins should be lower at the beginning of the treatment, since dangerous hypokalemia may occur (it is advised that potassium should be watched closely for the first several days of the therapy). It is also advised that folate acid be given to all patients with hemolytic anemia (increased cell turnover), as well as to pregnant women (with iron; starting at the fourth month of pregnancy and for several months thereafter).

Causes of Macrocytosis[a]

Megaloblastic Anemia
(suspect if MCV > 115)
    Vitamin B_{12} deficiency
    Folate acid deficiency

Increased Membrane Surface
    Liver disease (usually MCV < 110)
    Postsplenectomy

Reticulocytosis
(uncommon MCV > 115)
    Hemolysis
    Blood loss

Alcoholism[b]
(MCV 100–110)
    (in about 90% of patients)

Primary Hematologic Diseases
(usually MCV 100–110)
    Myelodysplastic syndrome
    Aplastic anemia
    Red cell aplasia
    Multiple myeloma
    Leukemia
    Myeloproliferative disease

Other Causes
    Drugs
    Hypothyroidism (50% of patients)
    Spurious (e.g., cold or warm agglutinins, marked leukocytosis, technical problems with counter, etc.)
    No obvious cause

Abbreviation: MCV, mean cell volume.
[a] Found in 15-20% of hospitalized patients
[b] The most common cause of macrocytosis in the U.S. (most patients are not anemic)

Causes of False-Negative and False-Positive Results of Vitamin B_{12} and Folic Acid Deficiency Tests

False-negative Results:
B_{12} deficiency exists (but serum levels normal/high)
    Myeloproliferative disorders
    Severe liver disease
    Transcobalamin (TC) II deficiency
    Laboratory error
    Transfusion
    Nitrous oxide inhalation
    Congenital cobalamin coenzyme deficiency

False-positive Results:
B_{12} deficiency does not exist (but serum levels low)
    Folate deficiency (10–60%)
    Pregnancy (B_{12} deficiency extremely rare)
    Vegan
    Oral contraceptive agents
    Deficiency of TC I/TC III
    Multiple myeloma (10–20%)
    Malignancy (5–10%)
    Aplastic anemia
    High-dose vitamin C
    Gastrectomy

False-negative Results:
Folate deficiency exists (but serum/RBC levels normal/high)
    Recent intake of folate (e.g., vegetables) (serum)
    Rare enzyme deficiencies
    Reticulocytosis (RBC folate)
    Blood transfusion (RBC folate)

False-positive Results:
Folate deficiency does not exist (but serum/RBC levels low)
    Recent intake of ethanol (serum)
    Recent lack of intake (serum)
    Vitamin B_{12} deficiency (serum/RBC folate)

Abbreviation: RBC, red blood cell.

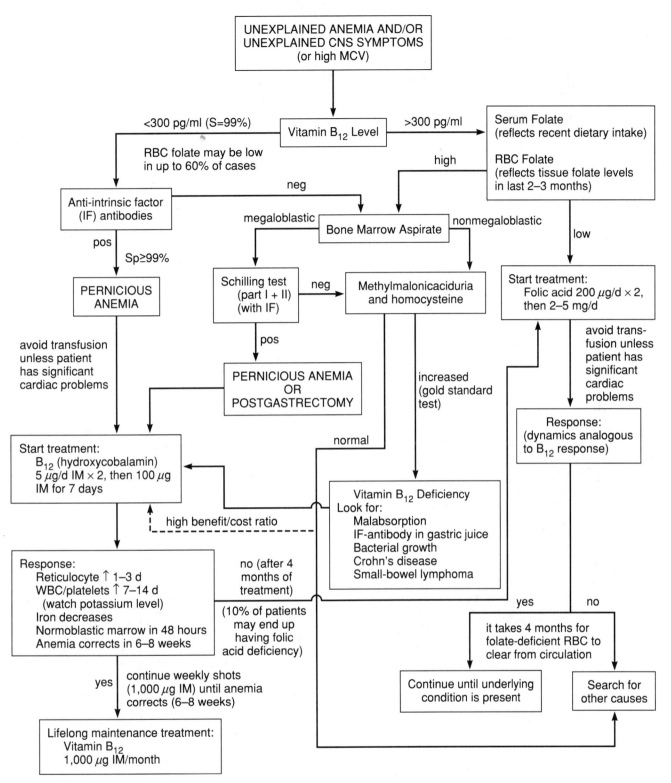

Fig. 6-1. Diagnostic and treatment strategies in megaloblastic anemia. Several elements were taken into consideration during the construction of this algorithm. First is the application of the *production rule*: if the patient has a low vitamin B$_{12}$ level and a positive anti-intrinsic factor antibody, then he/she suffers from pernicious anemia (some physicians will look for megaloblastic marrow as well). Since a relatively small number of people with low B$_{12}$ levels will be helped with this rule, a second element in the algorithm is to attempt to identify the cause of vitamin deficiency (*causal approach*) before replacement is started. Finally, elements of *cost/effectiveness* estimate dominate the clinical approach to megaloblastic anemia. Since diagnostic tests are far from being perfect, and the cost so small with benefit so high, many authors argue that every patient with unexplained anemia or CNS symptoms should be given a therapeutic trial with B$_{12}$ and/or folate.

Table 6.1. Operating Test Characteristics Used in Diagnosis of Megaloblastic Anemia

Diagnostic Test	Sensitivity (%)	Specificity (%)	Disease
B_{12} level:			
(<300 pg/ml)	99	70–80 (?)	B_{12} deficiency
(<200 pg/ml)	90–95	>95 (?)	B_{12} deficiency
Folate level	70–90 (?)	>90 (?)	Folate acid deficiency
RBC folate	>90 (?)	50–60	Folate acid deficiency
MCV > 130	5–10 (?)	100	B_{12} deficiency/folate acid deficiency
MCV > 105	11	95	B_{12} deficiency/folate acid deficiency
MCV > 95	62	82	B_{12} deficiency/folate acid deficiency
RDW > 15	54	51	B_{12} deficiency/folate acid deficiency
Hypersegmented neutrophils (5 cells with 5 lobes or 1 cell with 6 lobes)	91–95	77	B_{12} deficiency/folate acid deficiency
Anti-intrinsic factor antibody	50–60	>99	Pernicious anemia
Antiparietal antibody	90	50	Pernicious anemia
Achlorhydria	100	30–50 (?)	Pernicious anemia
Methylmalonic acid (M)[a]	96	96	B_{12} deficiency
Total homocysteine (H)	98	96	B_{12} deficiency
M + H	77	92	Response to B_{12} treatment
Megaloblastic marrow	98–100	95–100	B_{12} deficiency/folate acid deficiency
Schilling test (stage I and II)	25–85	86	Pernicious Anemia

[a] Considered a gold standard test

Suggested Readings

Allen RH, Stabler SP, Savage DG, Lindenbaum J: Diagnosis of cobalamin deficiency I : usefulness of serum methylmalonic acid and total homocysteine concentrations. Am J Hematol 34:90, 1990

Carmel R, Johnson CS: Racial patterns in pernicious anemia. Early age at onset and increased frequency of intrinsic-factor antibody in black women. N Engl J Med 298:647, 1978

Clementz GL, Schade SG: The spectrum of vitamin B_{12} deficiency. Am Fam Physician 41:150, 1990

Lindebaum J, Healton EB, Savage D, et al.: Neuropsychiatric disorders caused by cobalamin deficiency in the absence of anemia or macrocytosis. N Engl J Med 318:1720, 1988

Lindenbaum J, Savage DG, Stabler SP, Allen RH: Diagnosis of cobalamin deficiency II : relative sensitivities of serum cobalamin, methylmalonic acid and total homocysteine. Am J Hematol 34:99, 1990

McGrath K: Treatment of anaemia caused by iron, vitamin B_{12}, or folate deficiency. Med J Aust 151:693, 1989

7 | Aplastic Anemia

Aplastic anemia (AA) is a disease characterized by pancytopenia and hypocellular (or fatty) marrow. It is a rather rare disorder, with an annual incidence of about 2–6 per million population. In about 50% of these cases, the etiology is unknown ("idiopathic AA"). The second leading cause of AA is drug and chemical use. Based upon the severity of disease, AA can be considered as a *severe* or *moderate* disease. *Severe AA* is characterized by any two of the following blood criteria along with the presence of either marrow criteria: *blood criteria*: neutrophils <500/mm^3, platelets <20,000/mm^3, corrected reticulocytes <1%; *marrow criteria*: severe hypocellularity (<25%) or moderate cellularity (<50%) with less than 30% of hematopoietic cells. *Moderate AA* is defined as the failure to meet criteria for severe disease but with at least two of three blood counts decreased (reticulocytes <40,000/mm^3, platelets <40,000/mm^3, neutrophils <1,500/mm^3) with hypocellular marrow biopsy. If left untreated, 80–90% of patients with severe AA will die within a year. These patients die from infections (immunocompromised patients) or bleeding. The prognosis for patients with moderate AA is considerably better, although many patients will die of complications of pancytopenia or transfusion-related hemosiderosis. Prognostic systems have been developed and, in general, may be used to try to individualize treatment in particular patients. Two such systems are shown in the box below. Overall, age and level of granulocytopenia are the two most important prognostic determinants.

The treatment strategy of AA is based on consideration of the severity of the disease (i.e., a high probability of demise), data on the response rate to different kinds of treatment options, and the natural history of disease. Probabilistic aspects of clinical reasoning, as reflected by benefit/risk estimates, highly dominates clinical strategies in AA. Patients with severe AA should be treated immediately. Of those patients who die, the majority will die during the first 4 months and/or during the first two years (approximately 60%).

The natural history of the disease is characterized by the development of late hematologic complications, such as acute leukemia, paroxysmal nocturnal hemoglobinuria (PNH), etc. Interestingly, this incidence has risen from 5–15% to more than 57% in those patients treated with immunosuppressive therapy; these factors should be taken into account when treatment is planned.

Initially, supportive therapy is of utmost importance, and early institution of antibiotics is critical in these patients (see Chapter 30 for the treatment of immunocompromised patients). Platelets should be kept >20,000/mm^3. Granulocyte-macrophage colony-stimulating factors (GM–CSF), interleukin 3 (IL–3) and other growth factors will play an increasingly significant role during treatment of the aplastic phase of the disease.

The treatment of choice for *young patients* (<20 year old) with an HLA-compatible donor is bone-marrow transplantation (BMT). A candidate for BMT, if not transfused, has a long-term survival rate of over 75–80%, as compared with 40–65% for previously transfused patients. Therefore, if possible, one should avoid transfusion in BMT candidates.

The second line of treatment for patients with AA

Prognostic Systems in Aplastic Anemia

Data from Lynch et al.: (Blood 45:517, 1975)

$C = -0.01796(B) + 0.01272(S) - 0.00008(OFV) - 0.00359(R) - 0.000002(N) - 0.00018(P) + 0.00046(NM)$

Where:
- B = bleeding at onset of symptoms (0–present; 1–absent)
- S = sex (1–female, 2–male)
- OFV = interval between onset of symptoms and first clinic visit in months
- R = corrected initial reticulocyte count (in %)
- N = neutrophil count (cells/μl)
- P = initial platelet concentration (thousands/mm³)
- NM = percentage of nonmyeloid cells in initial marrow aspirate

If C > .041 patient, there is a 91% probability he/she will die within 4 months.[a]

If C < 0 patient, there is an 81% probability he/she will survive.[b]

Data from Najean Y, et al.: (Am J Med 67:564, 1979)

$PMI = .544A + .027B - .416C - .209D + .024E + .134F + .053G$

Where:
- A = % of myeloid cells in the bone marrow
- B = reticulocyte count (10^9/L)
- C = hemorrhagic symptoms (1–absent, 2–moderate, 3–severe)
- D = sex (1–male, 2–female)
- E = granulocytes (10^6/L)
- F = platelet count (10^9/L)
- G = delay between first symptoms and clinic visit (months)

If PMI > 75, patient will survive.
If PMI < 25, there is >60% of death probability.[c]

[a] sensitivity of the index—75%
[b] Sensitivity of the index—95%
[c] Overall predictive value is about 73%

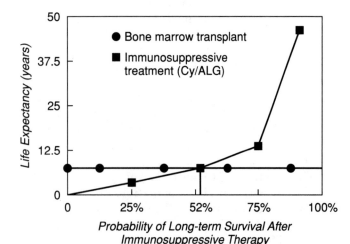

Fig. 7-1. Decision analysis of the treatment choice in patients with aplastic anemia aged 20–45. It can be seen that bone marrow transplantation (BMT) is the preferred option if long-term survival of patients treated with immunosuppressive therapy (IST) is less than 52%. Data indicate that development of late hematologic clonal disorders may be as high as 58% in patients treated with IST, with 26% developing MDS or acute leukemia. Late hematologic complications apparently do not develop in those patients treated with BMT.

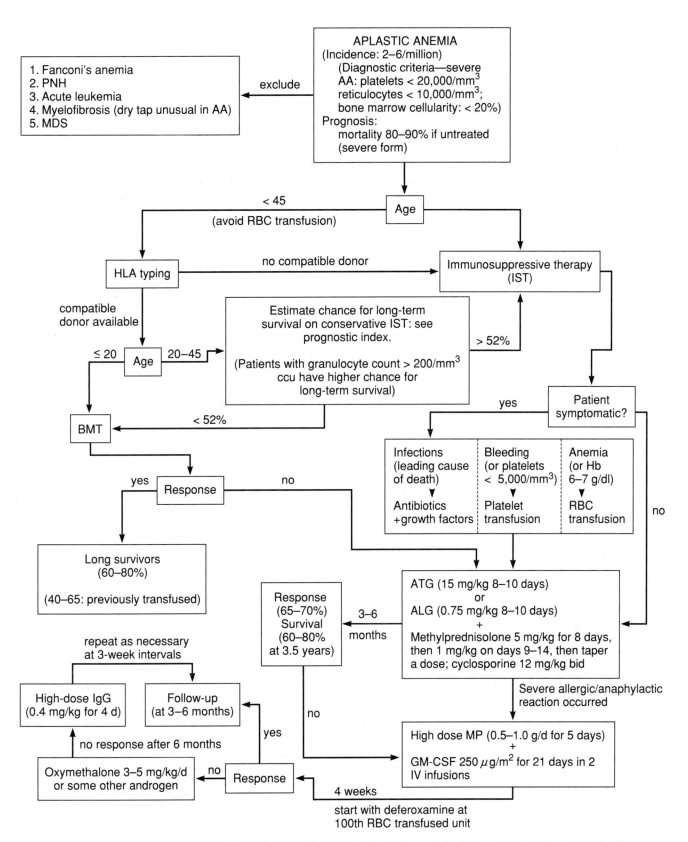

Fig. 7-2. Treatment strategy for patients with aplastic anemia (AA). Note that *probabilistic aspects* of clinical reasoning, as reflected in benefit/risk estimates, highly dominates clinical strategies in aplastic anemia. The major factors that the clinician has to take into consideration are prediction of the natural course of disease and probabilities of the response to the various forms of treatment, along with its associated risks (see also the second box in this chapter).

Practical Issues with Immunosuppressive Therapy in Aplastic Anemia

Shorter intervals of treatment with *antithymocyte globulin* (ATG) (10 days) are probably as efficacious as longer therapy (28 days). Although ATG does not seem to influence death-outcome in moderate AA, as compared with androgen therapy, about 30% of patients are transfusion independent in a 3 month period, as compared with virtually 0 in an androgen treated group. ATG can cause severe anaphylactic and allergic reactions. Serum sickness is described in about 47% of patients. Because of this, skin testing with 0.1 ml of 1 : 1,000 dilution of ATG in saline should be done before treatment with ATG. A severe local reaction (>.5 cm induration or erythema) or an immediate systemic reaction warrant exclusion from treatment. The usual way of administering ATG is to give *methylprednisone* (MP) (40 mg) with the daily dose (15 mg/kg) of ATG, diluted in 500 ml of physiologic saline. ATG is then given as an infusion over 4–5 hours through a microaggregate filter. The rest of the total daily dose of *prednisone* (1 mg/kg) is given orally. Antihistamines and meperidine are usually given for allergic symptoms.

Antilymphocyte globulin (ALG) is usually given as a slow infusion (8–12 h) in doses of 0.75 ml/kg for 8 consecutive days. In one protocol, MP was given in a single oral or IV dose of 5 mg/kg on days 1–8, then in a dose of 1 mg/kg on days 9–14, then tapering the dose over the next 14 days.

Cyclosporine is usually given orally twice a day in a dose of 12 mg/kg/day (adults). Doses are usually adjusted to achieve blood levels between 200–500 μg/L. Cyclosporine levels are usually determined at 2 week intervals. Interestingly, there is no significant correlation between cyclosporine blood levels and toxicity. Toxicity typically develops between 3 weeks and 3 months. Major adverse effects are reflected in liver toxicity. When transaminases are up, the clinician should stop therapy for 1–4 days and resolve treatment with a lower dose. If this does not help, therapy should be stopped.

Supportive care is of utmost importance. Selective gut decontamination with antibiotics, aggressive treatment with broad spectrum antibiotics and/or amphotericin-B at the first sign of infection, the use of prophylactic platelets transfusions (especially during the first 10 days to counter the antiplatelet effect of ALG/ATG), and application of growth factors should be rigorously pursued (see Chapter 30).

is immunosuppressive therapy (IST) with antithymocyte or antilymphocyte globulin (ATG or ALG) and/or cyclosporine. Although response rates as high as 85% have been reported, the true response rate to ATG seems to be between 40–60%. An analysis of data from the European registry indicated that for patients older than 20 years with moderately severe AA (those patients with 200–500 granulocytes/mm³), IST may be a superior form of therapy. However, given the increased risk of a clonal disorder after IST, but not after BMT, BMT can still be the preferred option for patients between 20–45 years of age, if estimated long-term survival after IST is less than 52% (Fig. 7-1). One should be aware that *complete* normalization of the blood count with any form of therapy is not usual. Long-term follow-up indicates that after 10 years, 85% of patients had a normal blood cell count, 80% had normal neutrophils, and 66% a normal platelet count. Late spontaneous improvements are also possible.

Details of a diagnostic and treatment outline are shown in Figure 7-2 and the box opposite.

Suggested Readings

Bacigalupo A, Hows J, Gluckman E, et al.: Bone marrow transplantation (BMT) versus immunosuppression for the treatment of severe aplastic anaemia (SAA): a report of the EBMT SAA working party. Br J Haematol 70:177, 1988

Bodenstein H: Successful treatment of aplastic anemia with high-dose immunoglobulin. N Engl J Med 324:1368 (letter), 1991

Frickhofen N, Kaltwasser JP, Schrezenmeier H, et al.: Treatment of aplastic anemia with antilymphocyte globulin and methylprednisolone with or without cyclosporine. N Engl J Med 324:1297, 1991

Moore MAS, Castro-Malaspina H: Immunosuppression in aplastic anemia—postponing inevitable. N Engl J Med 324:1358, 1991

Najean Y, Haguenauer O: Long-term (5–20 years) evolution of nongrafted aplastic anemia. Blood 76:2222, 1990

Tichelli A, Gratwohl A, Wursch A, et al.: Late haematological complications in severe anaemia. Br J Haematol 69:413, 1988

Young N, Griffith P, Brittain E, et al.: A multicenter trial of antithymocyte globulin in aplastic anemia amd related diseases. Blood 72:1861, 1988

8 | Hemolytic Anemia: Diagnostic Approach

The diagnostic approach to *hemolytic anemia* is traditionally built upon understanding the physiology of hematopoiesis; in the case of hemolysis, marrow can compensate for shortened red blood cell (RBC) survival. This in turn can be clinically detected by an increase in the reticulocyte count (see box below). Hemolysis itself can be caused by *immune mediated processes* (e.g., autoimmune hemolytic anemia), *defects in RBC membrane* (e.g., hereditary spherocytosis), *derangements in RBC enzyme machinery* (e.g., G-6-PD deficiency), *fault in the synthesis of hemoglobin molecules* (e.g., thalassemia or sickle cell disease), or *a mechanical disruption of erythrocytes* (e.g., microangiopathic hemolytic anemia). A useful production rule for the clinical workup of hemolytic anemia is based upon positivity of the *Coombs test* (see box). Still another production rule can be derived (production rule No. 3 in box), because tests for the detection of hemolysis are far from perfect (see Table 8-1 for summary of receiver operating characteristic (ROC) data on the most common tests used in detection of hemolysis).

The only tests that allow a distinction between *intravascular* and *extravascular hemolysis* (reticuloendothelial cell hemolysis) are free plasma hemoglobin and hemoglobinuria/hemosiderinuria. The latter is usually associated with complement-activation.

Due to the rarity of conditions, and many false-positives and false-negatives in assays of enzyme activities, some authors recommend that studies of RBC enzymopathies be done when all previous investigations have been completed. Others would leave testing for paroxysmal nocturnal hemoglobinuria (PNH) at the end of clinical workup. See Figure 8-1 for general workup of hemolytic anemia.

Production Rules for Workup of Hemolytic Anemia

1. *If* anemia is present and reticulocyte count[a] is increased, *then* suspect hemolytic anemia *and* order Coombs test.

2. *If* Coombs test is positive, *then* consider autoimmune hemolytic anemia (AIHA), *or else* suspect intracorpuscular red blood cell (RBC) defects or microangiopathic hemolytic anemia (MAHA) (Fig. 8-1).

3, *If* RBC drops *and* bleeding and overhydration is excluded, *then* suspect hemolysis.

4. *If* patient with condition known to cause hemolysis develops further drop in hemoglobin/hematocrit, *then* suspect *(1) aplastic crisis* (fall in reticulocyte count), *(2) hemolytic crisis* (increase in reticulocyte count), *(3) megaloblastic crisis*.

---

[a] Note the so-called *correct* reticulocyte count provides a different type of information than the *raw* reticulocyte count, and does not mean that a raw count is a wrong count. The corrected count provides evidence concerning red cell *production* (same information is provided by absolute reticulocyte count); a raw count, on the other hand, is an index of the red cell *life span*.

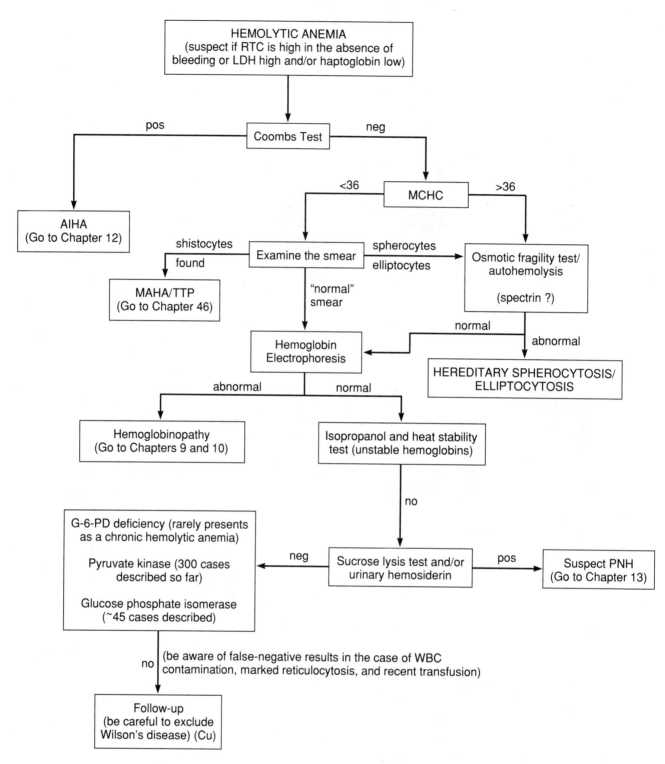

Fig. 8-1. Diagnostic approach to hemolytic anemia. An approach is derived from sets of production rules based upon an understanding of the pathophysiology of hemolytic disease (see box above) (*causal reasoning*), an assumption that mean cell hemoglobin concentration (MCHC), as a very specific test for hereditary spherocytosis (HS), is a more readily available test than smear examination (*principle of availability and representative heuristic*), and that HS is the most common Coombs negative hemolytic anemia (*probabilistic reasoning*). Note that routine diagnostic tests for hemolysis are far from perfect (Table 8-1), and that repeated tests will be needed to establish the hemolytic process (in order to increase specificity of tests). Note also a slightly different approach than in Figure 3-2 testing: it is not clear which is more cost-effective—to test for paroxysmal nocturnal hemoglobinuria (PNH) or for RBC-enzymopathies first.

Table 8-1. Operating Test Characteristics Used in Diagnosis of Hemolytic Anemia[a]

Diagnostic Test	Sensitivity (%)	Specificity (%)	Disease
History	75–100	?	HS, HE
Reticulocyte count[b]	62–90	99 (if >10%)	Hemolysis
Coombs test (anti-IgG only)	32	100	AIHA[b]
Coombs test (all reagents)	96–98	92	AIHA
MCHC	50	95–100	HS
Spherocytosis	95–100	90 (?)	HS
Splenomegaly	80–100	?	HS
Hb electrophoresis	95	>95 (?)	β-thalassemia
Haptoglobin (H) (<25 mg/dl)	83	96	Hemolysis
LDH (total) (high)	83	61	Hemolysis
LDH (isoenzymes)	58	93	Hemolysis
H+LDH (series testing)	50	100	Hemolysis
H+LDH (parallel testing)	92	89	Hemolysis
Hemosiderin (urine)	100	?	Intravascular Hemolysis (PNH)
MCV < 80 + RBC count increased	75	97	Thalassemia syndromes

Abbreviations: HS, hereditary spherocytosis; HE, hereditary elliptocytosis; MCHC, mean cell hemoglobin concentration; AIHA, autoimmune hemolytic anemia; PNH, paroxysmal nocturnal hemoglobinuria; MCV, mean cell volume; RBC, red blood cell; LDH, lactate dehydrogenase.
[a] Red blood cell (RBC) survival study with Cr^{51} is considered a gold standard test.
[b] For value of approximately 2.5%, predictive value for hemolytic disease is 38% only.

Suggested Readings

Crosby HW: Reticulocyte count. Arch Intern Med 141:1747, 1981

Friedman EW: Reticulocyte counts: how to use them, what they mean. Diag Med July:29, 1984

Galen RS: Application of the predictive value model in the analysis of test effectiveness. Clin Lab Med 2:685, 1982

Marchand A, Galen S, Van Lente F: The predictive value of serum haptoglobin in hemolytic disease. JAMA 243:1909, 1980

Palek J, Lambert S: Genetics of the red cell membrane. Semin Hematol 27:290, 1990

Petz LD, Garratty G: Acquired Immune Hemolytic Anemia. Churchill Livingstone, New York, 1980

Zanella A, Colombo B, Rossi F, et al.: Congenital nonspherocytic haemolytic anemias. Haematologica 74:387, 1989

9 | Thalassemia Syndromes

Thalassemia is the most common genetic disorder of man. α- and β-thalassemia together represent the most common anemias (Fig. 3-1). Reduction or deletion of alpha globin synthesis from 1–4 alpha genes on chromosome 16 will cause *alpha-thalassemia*, and a reduction of or absent beta globin synthesis from 1–2 beta genes on chromosome 11 will lead to *beta-thalassemia*. About 30% of black Americans are silent carriers for α-thalassemia. The incidence of the α-thalassemia trait (minor) is about 3% in black Americans, and 1–15% in the Mediterranean area. This incidence is even higher among the south Asian population: 5–40% (up to 80% of the population in some parts of New Guinea have the α-thalassemia trait). In Southeast Asia, the prevalence of β-thalassemia ranges between 10–15%, and is similar in other affected parts of the world. Fortunately, the majority of forms of thalassemia produce no clinical problems; the total number of *severe* cases of thalassemia in the U.S. is probably between 700 and 1,000.

The high incidence and prevalence of disease dictates a clinical approach to thalassemia. Prevention of a severe homozygous condition (which may occur if a baby is born to 2 heterozygous parents) via genetic counseling and antenatal detection with gene probes will ultimately be the treatment of choice. This decision is a very complex one, and depends not only on the medical aspects of the problem, but on ethical and legal views regarding abortion and the cost of medical therapy. In Greece and Italy, this approach has already decreased the prevalence of major thalassemia to less than 10% of the cases in the prescreening era.

What would be the *best* test to identify those people needing genetic counseling and/or further diagnostic workup? *Microcytosis* is a virtually 100% sensitive test for thalassemia (a minority of silent carriers may have a normal mean cell volume, or MCV), but it is not a specific test. Microcytosis and/ or mild microcytic anemia may create clinical problems because of confusion with iron deficiency anemia or other conditions that may be characterized by low MCV (Fig. 9-1). An elevated red blood cell (RBC) count with low MCV is 75% sensitive and 97% specific for thalassemia syndromes. A further diagnosis of thalassemia syndromes will require *electrophoresis of the hemoglobin*, which is a 95% sensitive test for the detection of increased levels of hemoglobin A_2; together with the elevation of hemoglobin F, it serves to diagnose β-thalassemia. In thalassemia minor these elevations are mild, with the majority of hemoglobin (>90%) still being hemoglobin A. In thalassemia major, hemoglobin A is absent and hemoglobin F present in concentrations > 50% (see Fig. 9-1 for a diagnostic approach to thalassemia syndromes). Milder forms of α-thalassemia can be demonstrated only with the use of sophisticated and not readily available tests of globin-chain synthesis and globin-gene analysis, using molecular biology techniques with DNA probes or polymerase chain reaction techniques. A diagnosis of α-thalassemia (type 1 and 2), therefore, still remains largely a diagnosis of exclusion. When three alpha genes are deleted, hemoglobin H is formed and can be detected by hemoglobin electrophoresis, as well as hemoglobin Bart's, which occurs as a result of a 4 gene deletion. This latter condition is incompatible with life, and results in the death of the fetus in utero.

The majority of patients with thalassemia do not

need any treatment outside of genetic counseling. Iron deficiency is important to exclude, so that these individuals are not inadvertently given iron therapy. *Hemoglobin H disease* behaves much like unstable hemoglobins, producing *Heinz bodies* (usually after a splenectomy) and hemolysis when the patient is exposed to infections, drugs, and other oxidant stresses (much like patients with G-6-PD deficiency). These patients should, therefore, avoid these stresses. A splenectomy should be reserved for severe anemia, and transfusions should be used judiciously. Major therapeutic decisions in the treat-

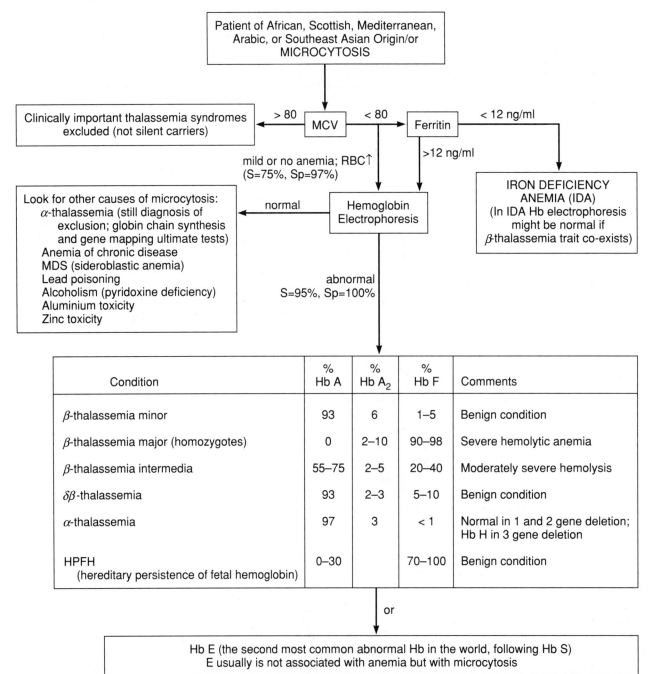

Condition	% Hb A	% Hb A_2	% Hb F	Comments
β-thalassemia minor	93	6	1–5	Benign condition
β-thalassemia major (homozygotes)	0	2–10	90–98	Severe hemolytic anemia
β-thalassemia intermedia	55–75	2–5	20–40	Moderately severe hemolysis
δβ-thalassemia	93	2–3	5–10	Benign condition
α-thalassemia	97	3	< 1	Normal in 1 and 2 gene deletion; Hb H in 3 gene deletion
HPFH (hereditary persistence of fetal hemoglobin)	0–30		70–100	Benign condition

or

Hb E (the second most common abnormal Hb in the world, following Hb S)
E usually is not associated with anemia but with microcytosis

Fig. 9-1. Diagnostic approach to thalassemia syndromes. Application of *principles of screening* for detection of high-prevalent disease is quite suitable here. (See also chapter 3, Fig. 3-1.) The approach will depend upon the estimate of pretest probability that a patient might have thalassemia, which is largely dependent on the patient's ethnic background. However, a clinically important diagnosis can virtually be excluded by a normal MCV, an inexpensive and highly sensitive test.

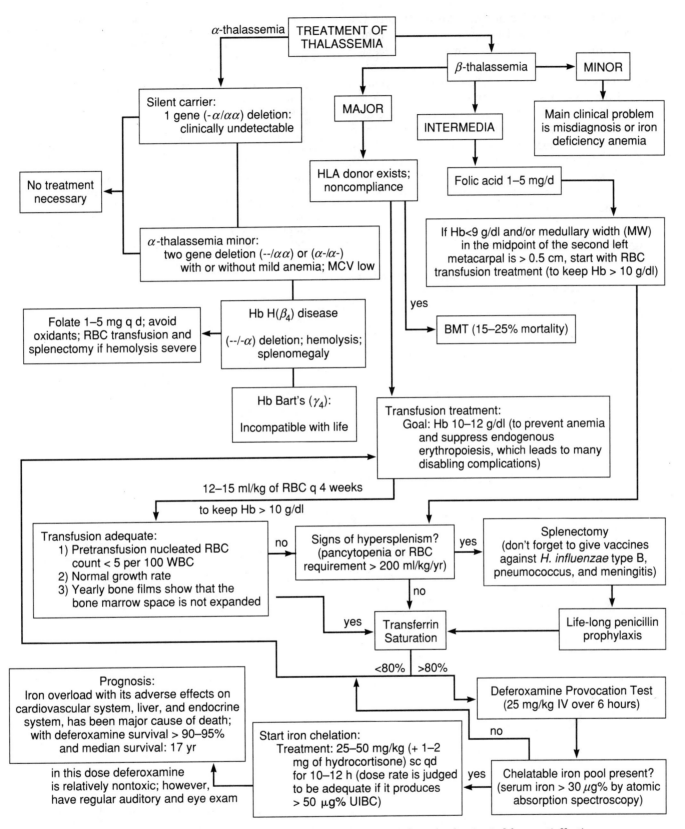

Fig. 9-2. Treatment of thalassemia syndromes. Decisions are largely dominated by *cost/effectiveness* issues. Since societal values are an important part of the decision making process, it is very difficult to present strategies of equal acceptance to all social groups.

ment of thalassemia major and intermedia are the initiation of transfusion therapy and chelation therapy, optimal timing of splenectomy, and indication for bone marrow transplantation. The *cost-effectiveness* element is the dominating decision component regarding these issues. On one hand, we have the option of not-widely-available bone marrow transplantation (BMT)—the only possible curative therapy, but with a mortality rate between 15–25%. On the other, there is the choice of a relatively nontoxic, but life-long nuisance—transfusion and chelation therapy. The outline of treatment for thalassemia is presented in Figure 9-2.

Suggested Readings

Anderson HM, Ranney HM: Southeast Asian immigrants: the new thalassemia in Americans. Semin Hematol 27:239, 1990

Fishleder AJ, Hoffman GC: Practical approach to detection of hemoglobinopathies: part I. The introduction and thalassemia syndromes. Lab Medicine 18:368, 1987

Fosburg MT, Nathan DG: Treatment of Cooley's anemia. Blood 76:435, 1990

Griner PF: Microcytic anemia. In Panzer RJ, Black ER, Griner PF (eds): Diagnostic Strategies for Common Medical Problems. American College of Physicians, Philadelphia, 1991

Kazazian HH: The thalassemia syndromes: molecular basis and prenatal diagnosis in 1990. Semin Hematol 27:209, 1990

Lucarelli G, Galimberti M, Polci P, et al.: Marrow transplantation in patients with advanced thalassemia. N Engl J Med 316:1050, 1987

Sbyrakis S, Karagiorga-Lagana M, Voskaki I, et al.: A simple index for initiating transfusion treatment in thalassemia intermedia. Br J Haematol 67:479, 1987

10 Sickle Cell Syndromes

Sickle cell disease (SCD) is the most common structural hemoglobinopathy in the U.S. It occurs almost exclusively among the black population, where 1 in 400 is homozygous for sickle cell hemoglobin (Hb SS), and 1 in 10 is an asymptomatic carrier for the disease (Hb AS). Another 2–3% of black Americans will inherit Hb C. Point mutation in the beta-globin gene (on chromosome 11) produces a change in the amino acid at position 6 (valine is changed to glutamic acid in the case of Hb S, but to lysine in the case of Hb C). In the case of Hb S, this in turn leads to easy polymerization in the deoxygenated state, resulting in the increment of blood viscosity and tissue hypoxia. Physiologic consequences of this sickling are manifested in the *vasoocclusive crisis* (micro- and macro-infarcts leading to painful crisis and organ damage), *anemia crisis* (due to severe hemolysis or aplastic crisis), and *impaired growth and development* with *increased susceptibility to infections*. This clinical manifestation relates to a homozygous condition (Hb SS), but not to a heterozygous state or sickle cell trait (Hb AS), which is essentially a benign condition. Interestingly, Hb C homozygotes are doing well clinically, and Hb S variants, such as coinheritance of the gene for β-, α-thalassemia, or Hb C, are clinically milder conditions than Hb SS disease (Table 10-1). A *production rule* is of help here: *If* the target cells are found and MCV is normal, *then* suspect Hb C disease. Similarly, *if* you suspect SCD, and microcytosis and/or splenomegaly is found, *then* suspect sickle (cell) thalassemia (S-thal) disease.

The diagnosis of sickle cell disease in adults is straightforward; a peripheral smear will usually show typical sickled erythrocytes. However, the gold standard test—an alkaline electrophoresis on cellulase acetate—does suffer from some false-positive results (S-thal, hereditary persistence of fetal hemoglobin (HPFH), Hb G, Hb D, Hb Lepore, unstable Hb Zurich—generally benign disorders, all may show similar migration capacity to Hb S). This is usually easy to discern through further testing (such as electrophoresis on citrate agar). Problems, however, may arise when an antenatal diagnosis is attempted.

Ironically, our deep understanding of events at the molecular level has not been paralleled by successful therapy. Treatment of sickle cell disease is still largely supportive, consisting of *hydration, oxygenation, and analgesia* (Fig. 10-1). Because of the supportive nature of treatment, the essential element

Table 10-1. Relative Clinical Severity of Various Structural Hemoglobinopathies

Type of Hemoglobin	Clinical Severity (0–4)
Hb SS, SO	4 (most severe)
Hb SC, SD	3
Hb CC	2
Hb OO, EE	1
Hb SG, SN, CO	0 (no clinical abnormality)

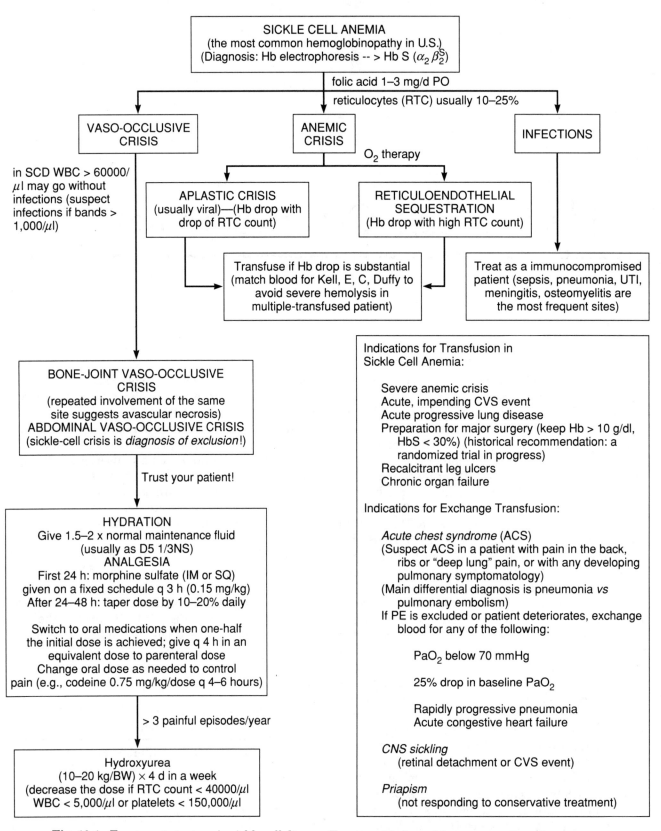

Fig. 10-1. Treatment strategy in sickle cell disease. Treatment is by and large supportive, since no cure is possible at this time. Clinical reasoning is dominated by *cost/effective* estimates regarding risk of therapeutic maneuvers, such as repeated transfusions and justification of the use of potentially toxic agents such as hydroxyurea (HU) (and/or BMT). Note an interesting *production rule* that may be applied when a patient is developing a crisis: *If* patient reports that a bout of pain represents something new and different from his/her usual crisis pain, *then* search for an infectious source more aggressively.

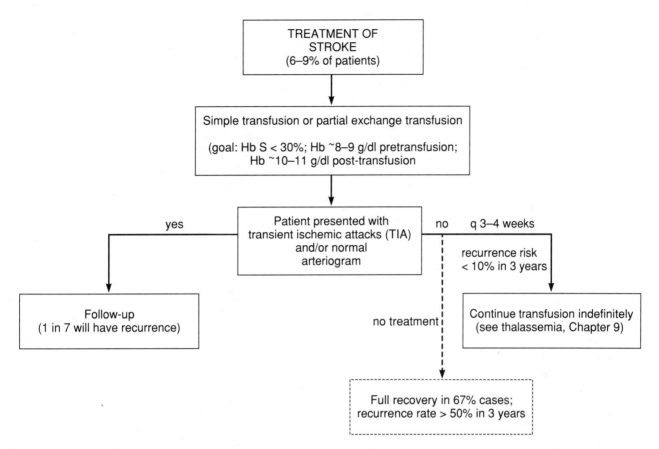

Fig. 10-2. Treatment approach to stroke in sickle cell disease in young patient. The suggested approach is highly *probabilistic* and represents a current interpretation of risk for stroke recurrence both with and without transfusion therapy. The quality of life and risks from long-standing transfusion therapy are not taken into consideration. The *comprehensive* decision *should* consider these factors. (Recent data indicate that noninvasive transcranial Doppler ultrasonography has S = 86% and Sp = 91% in predicting stroke in young people.)

of clinical reasoning in taking care of patients with SCD is the estimate of the *cost/benefit* of therapeutic maneuvers. Major therapeutic decisions are related to the use of blood transfusions. The majority of authors think that the long-term risks (isoimmunization, iron overload, HIV infection, hepatitis) associated with repeated transfusions outweigh its benefit, especially as patients tolerate anemia well between crises. Transfusions should be reserved for severe anemia crises (see Fig. 10-1 for indications for blood transfusion). Some authors advocate the use of chronic transfusions in the prevention of a stroke recurrence. The rationale for this is probabilistic. If Hb S is kept < 30%, recurrence risk is less than 10%, while in patients not enrolled in this program, a 3-year recurrence risk is greater than 50%. The optimal duration of this program is unresolved at this time, and some data indicate that life-long therapy (coupled with chelation therapy—see thal-

assemia, Chapter 9) would be indicated (a suggested approach to this problem is presented in Fig. 10-2).

The major problem in patients with SCD is infection. These patients should be treated vigorously with antibiotics as they are immunocompromised. Particular attention should be given to patients with chest or lung symptoms, because this is the leading cause of mortality in SCD. If pulmonary pathology is suspected, these patients should be hospitalized. Empirical treatment with IV cefuroxime (100 mg/kg/d) and erythromycin (if *Mycoplasma pneumonia* is suspected) is appropriate. (Interestingly, patients with SCD are the only group of patients who get *Salmonella osteomyelitis*, although *Staphylococcus* is the most common organism in the general population.) Remember that *a sickle cell crisis is a diagnosis of exclusion.* The most valuable piece of information used to make a distinction between a painful crisis and an infection may come from the

Table 10-2. Sickle Cell Comprehensive Care Outline

Type of Evaluation	Interval
Physical Examination:	
Younger than 6 months	Monthly
6 months to 1 year	Every 2 months
1 to 5 years	Every 3 months
Older than 5 years	Every 4 months
Social worker	Biannually
Social worker, home visit	Annually
School assessment	Annually
Genetic Counseling Services:	
Family studies	Initially
Counseling and education	Annually
Hematologic:	
CBC, reticulocyte count	Quarterly
Hemoglobin electrophoresis	Initially
Quantitative hemoglobin F	Initially
Kleihauer-Betke stain	Initially
Alpha gene mapping/haplotype analysis	Initially
Ferritin	Annually
Red cell alloantibodies	Baseline, before and after transfusion
Red cell phenotype	Initially
Liver-Gallbladder:	
Liver functions	Annually
Hepatitis antibody and antigen	Annually
Abdominal ultrasound	Biannually after age 10
Renal:	
BUN	Annually
Creatinine	Annually
Uric acid	Annually
UA	Annually
Cardiac:	
ECG	Biannually
Stress echocardiogram	Biannually
Pulmonary:	
Chest roentgenogram	Biannually after age 5
Pulmonary function tests	Biannually after age 5
Blood gases	Biannually after age 5
Dental Evaluation	Annually
Nutrition Assessment	Annually age 10 and up
Indirect Ophthalmologic Examination	Annually age 10 and up
Immunization Schedules:	
OPV/DPT/MMR and booster	Standard intervals
Pneumococcal vaccine	Age 1, 2, 6 years
H influenza vaccine	Age 2 months
Hepatitis B vaccine series	Initiate at 1 year
Influenza vaccine	Annually
Prophylactic penicillin	125 mg twice a day 3 months to 3 years
	250 mg twice a day after 3 years

Abbreviations: CBC, complete blood count; BUN, blood urea nitrogen; UA, urinalysis; ECG, electrocardiogram; OPV, poliovirus vaccine live oral; DPT, diptheria-pertussis-tetanus vaccine; MMR, measles-mumps-rubella vaccine.
(From Vichinsky: Semin Hematol 28:220, 1991, with permission.)

patient. A *production rule* for this is as follows: *If the patient reports that a bout of pain represents something new and different from his/her usual crisis pain, then* search for an infectious source more aggressively. Thought should be given to the possibility of an exchange transfusion as well (Fig. 10-1).

Studies of the natural history of disease show that about 40% of patients do not exhibit painful crises, and that about 5% of patients have 33% of all painful episodes (3–10 per year). There is also an inverse correlation between painful episodes and survival. On the other hand, the increase of fetal hemoglobin may have an ameliorating effect on the pain rate. In these patients, the use of agents such as hydroxyurea (HU) which would increase the level of Hb F, might be of benefit.

Modern comprehensive care has resulted in definitive prolongation of life expectancy for patients with SCD (Table 10-2). Eighty-five percent of patients survive 20 years (95% with Hb SC disease), with a projected survival of 60% at age 50 (80% for Hb SC disease). Longer survival, however, has introduced a shift in the clinical approach to these patients, making the management of chronic organ damage (stroke, renal failure, cardiovascular disease, chronic lung problems, aseptic hip necrosis) a primary issue. *Quality of life*, rather than mortality, then becomes the major determinant for the use of new experimental procedures such as bone marrow transplantation (BMT) and HU. BMT, with an estimated mortality risk of about 10–25%, has to be balanced against conventional therapy, the major

problem being how to identify those patients who will have a bad course of the disease (and would therefore be candidates for high-risk BMT) from those who do clinically well on conservative treatment. Currently, the majority of parents of young patients do not seem willing to accept the 15% mortality risk of the BMT procedure.

Suggested Readings

Adams R, McKie V, Nichols F, et al: The use of transcranial ultrasonography to predict stroke in sickle cell disease. N Engl J Med 326:605, 1992

Beutler E: Bone marrow transplantation for sickle cell anemia: summarizing comments. Semin Hematol 28:263, 1991

Francis RB, Johnson CS: Vascular occlusion in sickle cell disease: current concepts and unanswered questions. Blood 77:1405, 1991

Gilliland DG, Bridges KR: Management strategies for acute sickle cell crisis. Recognizing painful crisis, aplastic crisis, sickle lung syndrome. J Crit Illness October:25, 1988

Kodish E, Lantos J, Stocking C, et al.: Bone marrow transplantation for sickle cell disease. A study of parents' decisions. N Engl J Med 325:1349, 1991

Platt OS, Thorington BD, Brambilla DJ, et al.: Pain in sickle cell disease. Rates and risk factors. N Engl J Med 325:11, 1991

Rodgers GP, Dover GJ, Noguchi TC, et al.: Hematologic responses of patients with sickle cell disease to treatment with hydroxyurea. N Engl J Med 322:1037, 1990

Smith JA: What do we know about the clinical course of sickle cell disease. Semin Hematol 28:209, 1991

Vichinsky EP: Comprehensive care in sickle cell disease: its impact on morbidity and mortality. Semin Hematol 28:220, 1991

11 | Coombs-Negative Hemolytic Anemias

Hereditary Spherocytosis (HS)

HS is the most common defect of the red blood cell (RBC) membrane. It is associated with a quantitative deficiency of spectrin—and, in some cases, of ankyrin—and a deficiency of protein 4.2. It is inherited in an autosomal dominant fashion with a prevalence of about 1 in 5,000 patients of Northern European descent. Clinical clues to diagnosis are a strong positive family history (S = 75%), increased reticulocyte counts (S = 100%, usually in the range of 8–15%), jaundice, splenomegaly (S = 80–100%) and cholelithiasis (10–55%). The diagnosis requires a negative direct antiglobulin test and a positive osmotic fragility test, which is always abnormal (only 1–2% abnormal cells are needed to show positive). A radioimmunoassay test for spectrin and/or ankyrin will probably become the gold standard test for diagnosis (preliminary data suggest sensitivity and specificity close to 100%) and also the best predictor for response to a splenectomy. Major complications of HS are similar to other hemolytic anemias: *aplastic crisis* (hemoglobin (Hb) drop with reticulocytopenia), *hemolytic crises* (Hb drop with reticulocytosis) and *megaloblastic crises* in patients not taking folate.

A *splenectomy* is the treatment of choice for HS. The success of splenectomy should be judged after 3–6 months. Patients with spectrin levels above 70% achieve a normal blood count; those with levels between 40–70% have compensated hemolysis; and those below 40% improve but remain anemic. Overall, a splenectomy is largely curative, and life expectancy approaches normal. Splenectomy corrects anemia, but not spherocytosis.

Since a splenectomy is nearly always followed by a sustained thrombocytosis, low dose heparin (5,000 U q 12 h) is advised during the perioperative period, until the patient becomes fully ambulant. Because of the risk of pneumococcal sepsis, a splenectomy is not advised in children younger than 4 years. A major controversy exists as to whether a splenectomy should be performed in patients with mild hemolysis (hemoglobin less than 1 standard deviation (SD) from normal, and reticulocytosis less than 5%). The majority of authors believe these patients should be followed closely and given folic acid, as is recommended in all patients with hemolytic anemia.

Hereditary Elliptocytosis (HE)

HE is also a very common form of RBC membrane disorder (of spectrin self-association) with a prevalence rate in the U.S. of about 3–5 per 10,000 births. Main diagnostic features include a positive history (autosomal dominant disorder) and findings of elliptocytes on the smear (usually 25–95%). In normal people, elliptocytes are usually found in less than 5%; they can be found in many other disorders, such as iron deficiency anemia, myelodysplastic syndrome (MDS), myeloproliferative syndrome (MPS), etc., but rarely in percentages exceeding 60%. The major treatment decision is whether and when to perform a splenectomy. This will, by and large, depend on the severity of the hemolysis. In mild anemia (< 1 SD of Hb/hematocrit), a splenectomy will not be necessary (folate is recommended, however). Should the hemolysis be moderate to severe, a splenectomy is quite effective in improving the anemia.

Unstable Hemoglobin (US)

US can also present with spherocytosis on a peripheral smear, although typically a patient presents with a hemolytic crisis after exposure to infections or oxidative drugs (see box below). The reticulocytosis is often out of proportion to the severity of the anemia, because these patients often have increased O_2 affinity (something to consider in the differential diagnosis of methemoglobinemia, as well!) and the hemoglobin may be in the upper portion of normal range. Hemoglobin electrophoresis is usually normal. Isopropanol stability tests, heat stability tests and/or the presence of Heinz bodies in a patient with a positive family history (usually autosomal dominant inheritance), chronic hemolytic anemia, and splenomegaly are the diagnostic features of US. None of these features, however, is without false-positive results. Hb F, for example, can produce a false-positive isopropanol stability test. Fortunately, the course of this condition is benign, and all that is necessary is avoidance of oxidative drugs (particularly sulfa drugs) and the use of folic acid supplements. It is best to avoid a splenectomy until anemia becomes severe (see the rest of this chapter).

Nonspherocytic Hemolytic Anemias:
RBC Enzymopathies

Glucose-6-phosphate dehydrogenase (G-6-PD) deficiency is the most common enzymopathy of the pentose phosphate pathway responsible for generating NADPH, a coenzyme required for reduction of GSSG to GSH. Any hindrance to this pathway will greatly increase the risk of oxidant damage to the RBC. There are more than 400 G-6-PD mutants, and it has been estimated that more than 200 million people are deficient in this enzyme. The gene is carried on the X chromosome; hence, only males usually suffer from this condition (because of the high prevalence of this enzyme deficiency, it is not uncommon that a homozygous female may suffer from the disease as well).

The normal enzyme is denoted as *G-6-PD B*. Disease can manifest in three forms: *icterus neonatorum*, the most severe form, where exchange transfusion may be life-saving. A mild form of this deficiency, *G-6-PD A- variant*, is the most common type present in American blacks: about 11% of the black population (these patients have about 10% of residual enzyme activity). The severe form of the deficiency, *G-6-PD Mediterranean*, (enzyme activity is scarcely detectable in RBC) can be fatal, but fortunately produces anemia only under unusual circumstances. Patients with this form of defect may develop devastating consequences when exposed to fava beans (*favism*). Hemolysis in G-6-PD deficiency is typically *acute intravascular*, and *no hemolysis or anemia* exists when patients are not exposed to

Some Drugs and Chemicals That Induce Hemolysis in Persons with Unstable Hemoglobin and G-6-PD Deficiency	
Acetanilid	Niridazole
Doxorubicin	Nitrofurantoin
Furazolidone	Phenazopyridine
Methylene blue	Primaquine
Nalidixic acid	Sulfamethoxazole

Some Drugs and Chemicals That Can Safely Be Given in Therapeutic Doses to Persons With G-6-PD Deficiency Without Nonspherocytic Chronic Hemolytic Anemia	
Acetaminophen	Probenecid
Ascorbic acid	Procainamide
Aspirin	Pyrimethamine
Chloramphenicol	Quinidine
Chloroquine	Quinine
Colchicine	Streptomycin
Diphenhydramine	Sulfamethoxypuridazine
Isoniazid	Sulfisoxazole
Menadione sodium bisulfite	Trimethoprim
Phenacetin	Tripelnnamine
Phenylbutazone	Vitamin K
Phenytoin	

(Modified from Beutler: N Engl J Med 324:169, 1991, with permission.)

stress factors such as infections (being the most common precipitating factor) or oxidative drugs. There are, however, fortunately rare variants of G-6-PD that do produce chronic nonspherocytic hemolytic anemia and that do not respond to a splenectomy.

With so prevalent a disease, one of the major decisions would seem to be whether a screening program to detect asymptomatic patients should be undertaken. Since this disease is rarely of sufficient clinical severity to justify such a search, little is to be gained from these programs (tests should be ordered only if subsequent management will differ; see also Chapter 3). Therefore, the major approach is a preventive one (i.e., avoidance of drugs and chemicals that have oxidant characteristics—see box above), and treatment of intravascular crisis, should it occur (Fig. 11-1). In this setting, a diagnosis is made by measurement of G-6-PD activity in RBC. Classical Heinz bodies are present only in the acute phase and visible only with methyl violet. A *cyanate-ascorbate test* is the most useful screening test once hemolysis has occurred (reticulocyte may have normal G-6-PD activity, and thus produce false-negative results), or a G-6-PD tetrazolium cytochemical

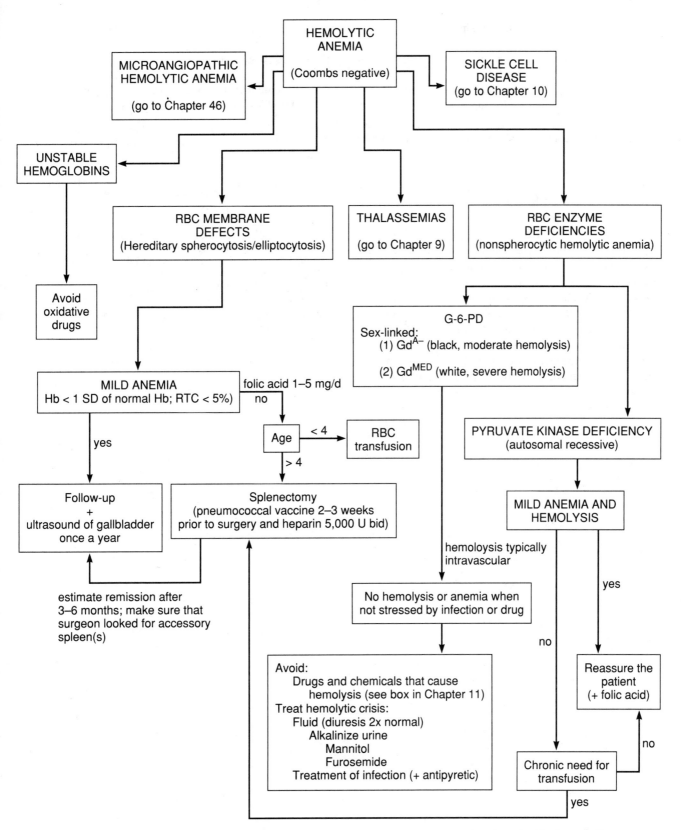

Fig. 11-1. Treatment of Coombs-negative hemolytic anemia (see text for further details). Understanding physiologic consequences of severe anemia and the vital role of the spleen in hemolysis dominates our reasoning in the treatment of HS/HE and pyruvate kinase deficiency anemia (*causal approach*). In G-6-PD deficiency, a low probability of severe cases of hemolysis (despite a high prevalence of disease) dictates a preventive approach (i.e., low-cost measures and aggressive treatment when severe hemolysis occurs, due to higher *cost/benefit* ratio in asymptomatic state).

test for the female heterozygous. A splenectomy is of little benefit.

Pyruvate kinase (PK) deficiency is the most common enzymopathy of the Embden-Meyerhof glycolytic pathway (>95%). So far, more than 300 cases have been described worldwide, with 65 occurring in Japan. Hemolysis in this condition is quite variable, ranging from transfusion-dependent anemia to mild, well-compensated hemolysis. Occasionally, elliptocytes may be found in the peripheral smear. A diagnosis, as in G-6-PD deficiency, is established by measuring red cell PK activity. In order to avoid false-negative results, an analysis should be run with substrate used at a low concentration and/or a supplement with determination of RBC 3-phosphoglycerate, which seems to be increased in PK deficiency. The treatment of choice is a splenectomy, which produces an increase in Hb 2–3 g/dl (20–30 g/L), and is accompanied by a high reticulocyte count (>40%) ("paradoxical reticulocytosis"). Again, the decision to perform a splenectomy is based upon the degree of anemia.

Suggested Readings

Agre P, Asimos A, Casella JF, et al.: Inheritance pattern and clinical response to splenectomy as a reflection of erythrocyte spectrin deficiency in hereditary spherocytosis. N Engl J Med 315:1579, 1986

Beutler E: Glucose-6-phosphate dehydrogenase deficiency. N Engl J Med 324:169, 1991

Beutler E: Hemoglobinopathies associated with unstable hemoglobin. In Williams WJ, et al. (eds): Hematology (4th Ed). McGraw-Hill, New York, 1990

Boyd AS: Hereditary spherocytosis. Am Fam Physician 39:167, 1989

Friedman EW, Williams JC, Van Hook L: Hereditary spherocytosis in elderly. Am J Med 84:513, 1988

Miwa, Fujii H: Pyruvate kinase deficiency. Clin Biochem 23:155, 1990

Tanaka KR, Zerez CR: Red cell enzymopathies of the glycolytic pathway. Semin Hematol 27:165, 1990

Valentine WN: Hemolytic anemias and erythrocyte enzymopathies. Ann Intern Med 103:245, 1985

12 | Autoimmune Hemolytic Anemias (Coombs-Positive)

Autoimmune hemolytic anemias (AIHA) comprise a group of disorders whose common characteristics are the presence of an autoantibody (-ies), which in turn causes short red blood cell (RBC) life. The approach to AIHA involves questions regarding (1) the type of autoantibodies (*warm* vs *cold*), and (2) the presence or absence of underlying disease (*idiopathic* vs *secondary AIHA*). (Fig. 12-1.)

The annual incidence of AIHA is estimated to be 1 case per 80,000 of the population. 70–80 percent of these cases are due to *warm-reacting autoantibodies* (WAHA), 10–20% are due to *cold agglutinin disease* (CAD), and 2–5% are due to *paroxysmal cold hemoglobinuria* (PCH). The incidence of idiopathic AIHA may vary from 20–80%. Lymphoproliferative disorders account for about half of the secondary cases of AIHA, of both warm and cold antibody types.

The cornerstone of diagnosis is a *positive Coombs antiglobulin test* in the presence of hemolysis. A positive *direct* Coombs test speaks for autoantibody mediated hemolysis, while a positive *indirect* Coombs test (in the absence of direct Coombs test) points to the presence of alloantibody (stimulated by prior transfusions or pregnancies). The Coombs test (best done on EDTA specimen) still has false-negative and false-positive rates in about 2–4% and 8% of all cases, respectively (see Table 3-1, Chapter 3). (If the test is done with IgG reagent only, sensitivity can drop to 32%, although specificity will be closer to 100%.) If agglutination is noted with a broad spectrum Coombs reagent, antisera reacting with a specific class of immunoglobulins or monospecific antisera against IgG, IgM, IgA or components of complement may be employed to further characterize the pattern of sensitization. Anti-IgG autoantibodies are found in about 90% of cases in WAHA; it is very unusual to have isolated IgA or IgM warm autoantibodies. A Coombs test is positive during hemolytic attacks of PCH; and a Coombs test done with anti-C3 or anti-C3dg is positive in CAD. Cold agglutinins are virtually always IgM; the serum titers are commonly 1:10,000 or higher, but they are not detected by the antiglobulin test because these proteins easily dissociate from RBCs during washing procedures. *Anti-I* is of predominant specificity in idiopathic CAD, but is seen in CAD secondary to mycoplasma pneumonia and lymphoma. *Anti-i* is seen in CAD associated with infectious mononucleosis. *Donath-Landsteiner antibody*, found in PCH, has a specificity for the P blood group antigen, and can be proven by incubation at 4°C, followed by warming at 37°C when complement-mediated intense hemolysis occurs. Intravascular hemolysis is typical in both CAD and PCH.

The treatment of an *underlying* cause is a logical strategy in the management of secondary AIHA; therefore, the prognosis obviously depends on the prognosis of the underlying disease. *Steroids* are the cornerstone of WAHA therapy, followed by a splenectomy (Fig. 12-2). Despite rather high initial responses to these modalities, actuarial survival at 10 years in idiopathic WAHA is reported to be 73% and, most recently, 80% at five years. Pulmonary emboli, infection (*do not forget to administer Pneumovax vaccine 2–3 weeks before splenectomy*), and severe anemia are the leading causes of death. Steroids and splenectomy have not been useful in CAD and PCH, although some data suggest that IV steroids may

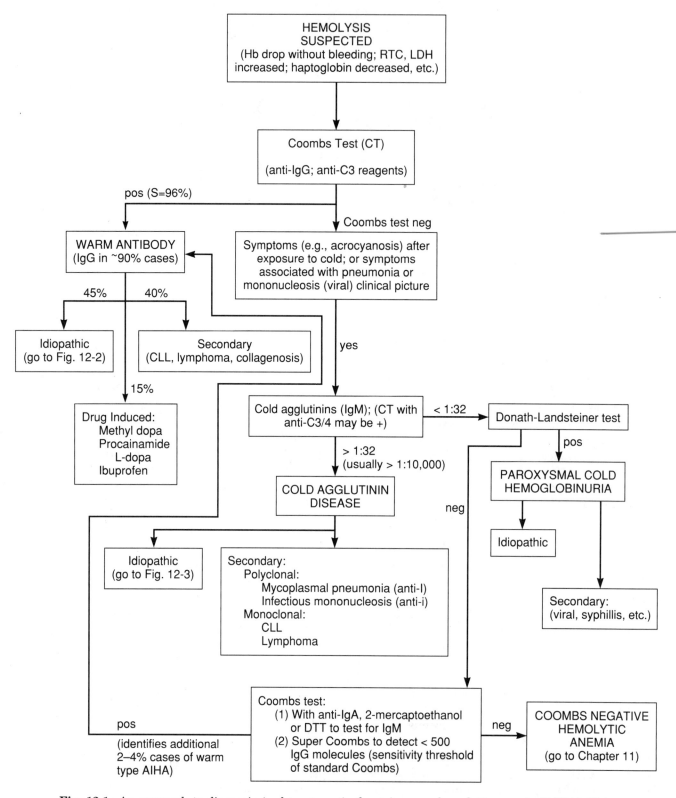

Fig. 12-1. An approach to diagnosis (and treatment) of autoimmune hemolytic anemia (AIHA). This approach is based upon the *production rule,* which is derived from the understanding of the pathophysiology of AIHA (i.e., that a positive Coombs test defines one set of disorders and a negative test defines a different set of conditions). Note that a Coombs test is not a perfect test, and that sensitivity and specificity vary depending on the type of reagent used. We propose initial testing with IgG and C3 reagents, which will detect 96% of all cases. It would be more cost-effective to detect those additional 4–5% cases with extra reagents after CAD and PCH are excluded.

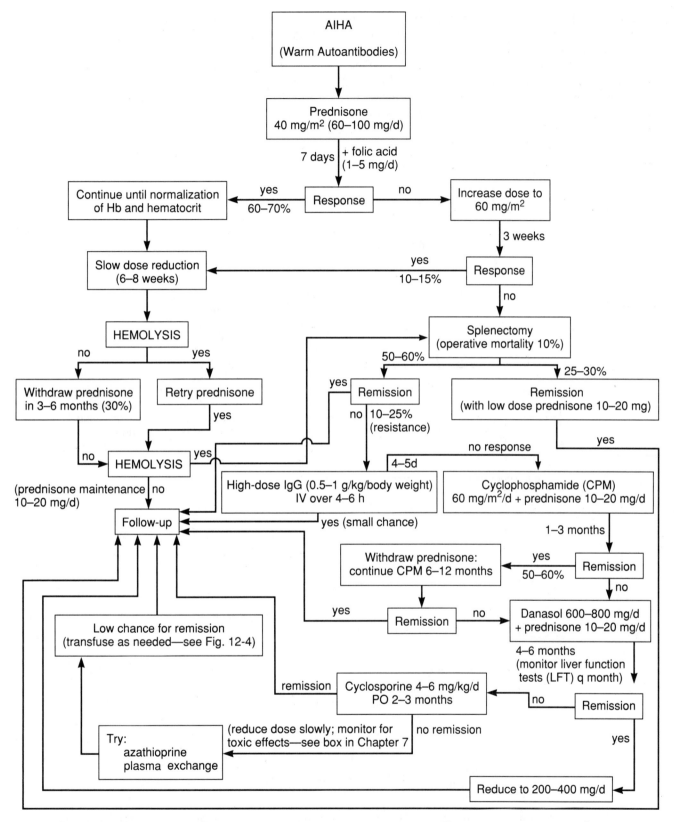

Fig. 12-2. Treatment of autoimmune hemolytic anemia (warm type). Treatment sequences are determined by estimates of the *probability* of the response to various modalities, and, to some extent, by higher benefit/cost ratio as well.

decrease complement-coated RBCs by the reticulo-endothelial system in CAD. Avoidance of cold may be all that is necessary for some patients suffering from CAD and PCH. In other CAD patients, chlorambucil or cyclophosphamide may be tried (Fig. 12-3), followed by plasmapheresis, or even α-interferon, according to one case report. Typically, postinfectious forms of CAD and PCH are rather self-limiting disorders, and patients with idiopathic forms of these diseases may survive for many years.

Drug-induced AHA is usually mild, and a direct antiglobulin test becomes negative after the drug is cleared from circulation. In some cases, such as an α-methlydopa drug, a positive direct antiglobulin test may remain so for months.

Occasionally, when symptoms of anemia are severe, patients with AIHA must be *transfused*. Transfusion of erythrocytes in AIHA presents two problems: (1) cross-matching, and (2) rapid in vivo destruction of RCBs. Transfused cells will be destroyed

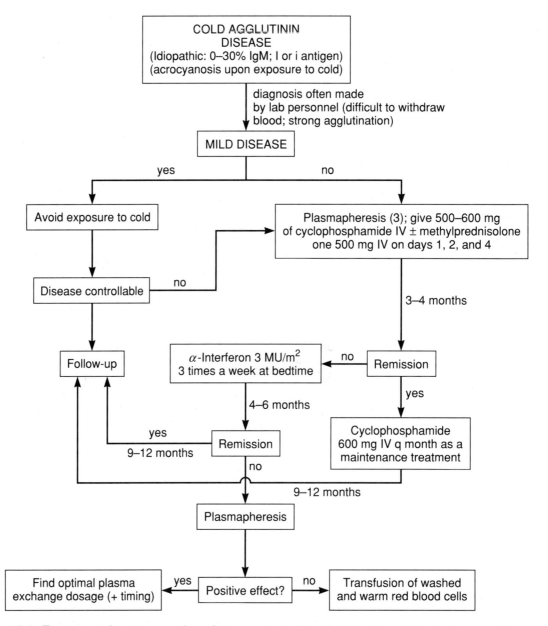

Fig. 12-3. Treatment of autoimmune hemolytic anemia (cold agglutinin disease). As in the case of warm type AIHA, treatment sequences are determined by estimates of the *probability* of the response to various modalities. However, because of the low incidence of this condition, the proposed estimates may be inaccurate, and the choice of other (alkylating) drugs may be equally correct.

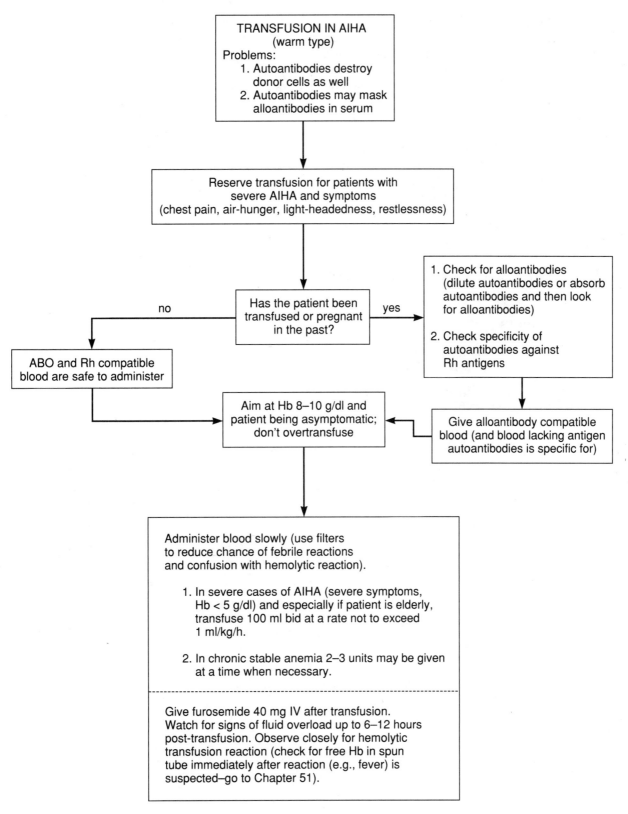

Fig. 12-4. A careful estimate of *risk/benefit* is the key in making a decision regarding the transfusion of patients with AIHA. A wrong decision—to transfuse or not to transfuse—can be as detrimental to the patient as no decision.

according to the kinetics of the first order—the more cells given, the more cells destroyed. This in turn can cause disseminated intravascular coagulation (DIC) and fatal embolic complications. Therefore, relatively smaller volumes of packed RBCs should be transfused. Transfused blood should also be *alloantibody compatible blood*, to avoid the danger of hemolytic transfusion reactions (Fig. 12-4). A number of methods are available to adsorb the autoantibody, which interferes with cross-matching, but it is of utmost importance to determine the Rh phenotype of a patient, along with a determination of other potent immunogenic RBC antigens (Kell, Duffy, etc.). Blood samples should be saved for future autoadsorption studies in order to facilitate locating the "right" blood. In CAD, it is important to prewarm the blood to body temperature before transfusion.

Suggested Readings

Ahn YS, Harrington WJ, Mylvaganam R, et al.: Danasol therapy for autoimmune hemolytic anemia. Ann Intern Med 102:298, 1985

Coon WW: Splenectomy in the treatment of hemolytic anemia. Arch Surg 120:625, 1985

Nydegger UE, Kazatchkine MD, Miescher PA: Immunopathologic and clinical features of hemolytic anemia due to cold agglutinins. Semin Hematol 28:66, 1991

O'Connor BM, Clifford JS, Lawrence WD, Logue GL: Alpha-interferon for severe cold agglutinin disease. Ann Intern Med 111:255, 1989

Omine M, Karasawa T, Maekawa T, et al.: Follow-up results of warm-type autoimmune hemolytic anemia: a study on 159 prospectively collected patients. Blood 76:43a, 1990

Petz LD: Red cell transfusion problems in immunohematological disease. Ann Rev Med 33:355, 1982

Silverstein MN, Gomes MR, Elveback LR, et al.: Idiopathic acquired hemolytic anemia. Survival in 118 cases. Arch Intern Med 129:85, 1972

13 | Paroxysmal Nocturnal Hemoglobinuria

Paroxysmal nocturnal hemoglobinuria (PNH) is an acquired stem cell disorder with an incidence of about 2 per million of the population. It is usually regarded as an *intravascular hemolytic disorder*, manifested through hemoglobinemia and hemoglobinuria, unusual venous thrombosis, and episodes of severe pain in the abdomen and back. This disease can also present with hypoplastic marrow and accompanying pancytopenia (platelets are low in about 80% of patients), leading to infections and bleeding. The hallmark of PNH is increased sensitivity of red blood cells (RBC) to complement-mediated lysis. This has been the basis for diagnosis of PNH for decades, with two tests usually performed to exclude disease (*sucrose lysis test*) and confirm disease (*Ham acid hemolysis test*), respectively. Although the sensitivity of the sucrose lysis test approaches 100%, false-negative results can still occur. *Hemosiderinuria* is almost always present in PNH, and its absence virtually excludes the disease (as much as 22 g of hemoglobin and 20 mg of iron as hemosiderin may be lost in a single day). PNH should still be confirmed by the highly specific Ham acid hemolysis test, which is *sine qua non* for the diagnosis of this disease and can be positive only in one other disease—HEMPAS (hereditary erythroblastic multinuclearity with an acidified lysis test). The disorders are easily distinguished on clinical grounds. Sensitivity of PNH to complement may be quantified, leading to classification of PNH: type I (normal sensitivity), type II (3–5 times as sensitive as normal cells), type III (10–15 times as sensitive as normal cells). Thresholds for lab detectability is 1%, but lysis > 5% is considered consistent with PNH.

Numerous proteins are deficient in PNH: leukocyte alkaline phosphatase (LAP) in white blood cells (WBC)—(the other condition where LAP is typically low is chronic myelocytic leukemia (CML), and occasionally myelodysplastic syndrome (MDS), idiopathic thrombocytopenic purpura (ITP), infectious mononucleosis, pernicious anemia, and congenital hypophosphatasia); acetylcholinesterase in RBC; decay accelerating factor (DAF or CD55) in all three cell lines; and also membrane inhibitor of reactive lysis (MIRL, or CD59), monocyte CD14, granulocytes CD24, CD67, etc. Monoclonal antibodies have been raised against these proteins and can serve as diagnostic tests, some of them appearing more sensitive than the Ham test. At pathogenic levels, it became apparent that post-translational defects in membrane anchoring proteins leads to increased susecptibility to complement-mediated hemolysis. A normal hematopoietic progenitor cell contains MIRL and DAF, which inhibit activation of the C3 part of the complement by the membrane-bound C3 convertase. When those proteins disappear during the hematopoietic maturation process, cells (RBC, granulocytes, platelets) become sensitive to the lytic effects of the complement. The abnormal clone appears to arise most commonly in a damaged marrow; many patients have a history of aplastic anemia prior to development of this disease.

PNH is a rare disease, which probably explains why 2–3 years is the average time to diagnosis. *PNH should be suspected in all patients with acquired chronic hemolytic conditions who are Coombs negative or who have unexplained pancytopenia* (see production rule in Table 3-2).

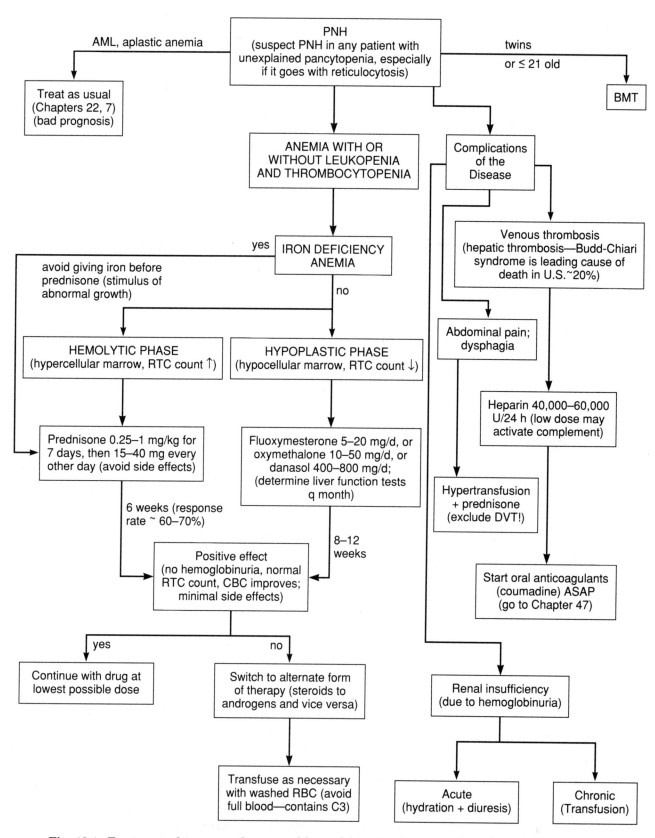

Fig. 13-1. Treatment of paroxysmal nocturnal hemoglobinuria. An approach is derived from the understanding of the natural course of disease (*physiologic model*), *probability of the response* to various forms of therapy (androgens, steroids, anticoagulants, BMT, etc.), and estimate of the *benefit/risk* for each form of therapy.

Therapy of PNH is supportive, and consists mainly of transfusions, antibiotics, and anticoagulants as required. The majority of physicians would transfuse patients with washed RBCs or frozen deglycerolized RBCs in order to provide blood without complement components. Androgen and glucocorticoids are commonly administered (Fig. 13-1). From the practical point of view, the physician should try to make a distinction between hemolytic and aplastic components of the disease. Bone marrow transplantation has been shown to be effective, although it is a risky method for the treatment of PNH.

The *prognosis* depends on complications. Hepatic thrombosis is a leading cause of death in this disease in both the U.S. and England, but hemorrhaging is the major cause of death in Japan. Thirty-year survival rate in one series was 57.5%. This prolonged survival speaks against bone marrow transplant (BMT) as an initial treatment of choice. However, median survival of PNH cases with an onset in childhood and adolescence is only 13.5 years. It can be argued that, in these cases, BMT may be the therapy of choice; risk/benefit estimates will dictate this decision. The development of acute leukemia is rare but well-documented. In this case, the prognosis is grave. Other patients may experience a chronic type of disease, waxing and waning for years. Details of the treatment outline are shown in Figure 13-1.

Suggested Readings

Fujioka S, Asai T: Prognostic features of paroxysmal nocturnal hemoglobinuria in Japan. Acta Haematol Jpn 52:1386, 1989

Rosse WF: Treatment of paroxysmal nocturnal hemoglobinuria. Blood 60:20, 1982

Rosse WF: Dr. Ham's test revisited. Blood 78:547, 1991

Rotoli B, Luzzatto L: Paroxysmal nocturnal hemoglobinuria. Semin Hematol 26:201, 1989

van der Schoot E, Huizinga TWJ, van Veer-Korthof ET, et al.: Deficiency of glycosylphosphatidylnositol-linked membrane glycoproteins of leukocytes in paroxysmal nocturnal hemoglobinuria, description of a new cytofluorometric assay. Blood 76:1853, 1990

Ware RE, Hall SE, Rose W: Paroxysmal nocturnal hemoglobinuria with onset in childhood and adolescence. N Engl J Med 325:991, 1991

14 Hereditary (Idiopathic) Hemochromatosis

Hereditary hemochromatosis is the most common iron-overload disorder, and is pathogenically related to the inherited tendency to absorb excessive amounts of iron from a normal diet. It is possibly the most common autosomal recessive disorder in Caucasians, with a carrier frequency estimated at about 1 in 10 individuals. This means at least 2–3 homozygous affected per 1,000 people. The affected gene is tightly linked to the human leukocyte antigen (HLA) locus on the short arm of chromosome 6.

The iron overload will, over time, result in the damage of vital organs. Liver cirrhosis (usually when iron concentration exceeds 2,000 μg iron/100 mg tissue), with hepatoma as a terminal event, is a typical characteristic of the disease. Other disease characteristics include failure of the heart, pancreas, and other endocrine glands, such as the anterior pituitary and endocrine pancreas. The patient may, therefore, present with hepatomegaly, ascites, cardiac heart failure and arrhythmias, arthritis, central nervous system (CNS) changes, loss of body hair, and gonadal dysfunction (impotence is very often an early sign of the disease). The classic advanced picture manifests with diabetes mellitus and skin hyperpigmentation due to melanin deposits: bronze diabetes*. The median time to diagnosis is 5 years in women and 8 years in men. Figure 14-1 shows the sequence of events in inherited hemochromatosis and their correlation with iron overload as measured by the serum ferritin (1 μg/L of ferritin corresponds to 7.5 mg of body iron in the absence of liver disease or inflammation).

Since this is a common disease, where effective treatment exists if instituted early enough, the major decisions in hemochromatosis cases are (1) early diagnosis (i.e., screening—family of the affected patient, and general population), and (2) early treatment (i.e., removal of iron before its toxic effects have started). An analysis of the cost-effectiveness of screening the general population has not been performed and, at this time, is regarded as investigational. Screening of family members in the proband case is obligatory, however.

A diagnosis is usually first suspected on the accidental finding of high iron in the blood. The most sensitive test is the combination of transferrin saturation (TS) with ferritin (F) (S = 94%). The most specific test is serum ferritin (Sp = 95%). (Interestingly, TS has better specificity than F when the test is applied in the screening of the general population.) To reduce false-positive results, fasting blood samples should be obtained on at least three occasions over a 1–3 month period. A liver biopsy is required to confirm the diagnosis (marrow iron stores are not increased). Usually, more than 50% of the hepatocytes are involved. HLA typing plays no role in the diagnosis of sporadic cases of hemochromatosis. However, it is indicated in family members when a diagnosis of hemochromatosis is already established, since there is at least a 25% chance of their being homozygous for the disease. Figure 14-2 shows an algorithm for the *diagnosis* of hemochromatosis.

The treatment of choice is still lifelong phlebotomy

---

* In more recent studies, found in only 8% of patients.

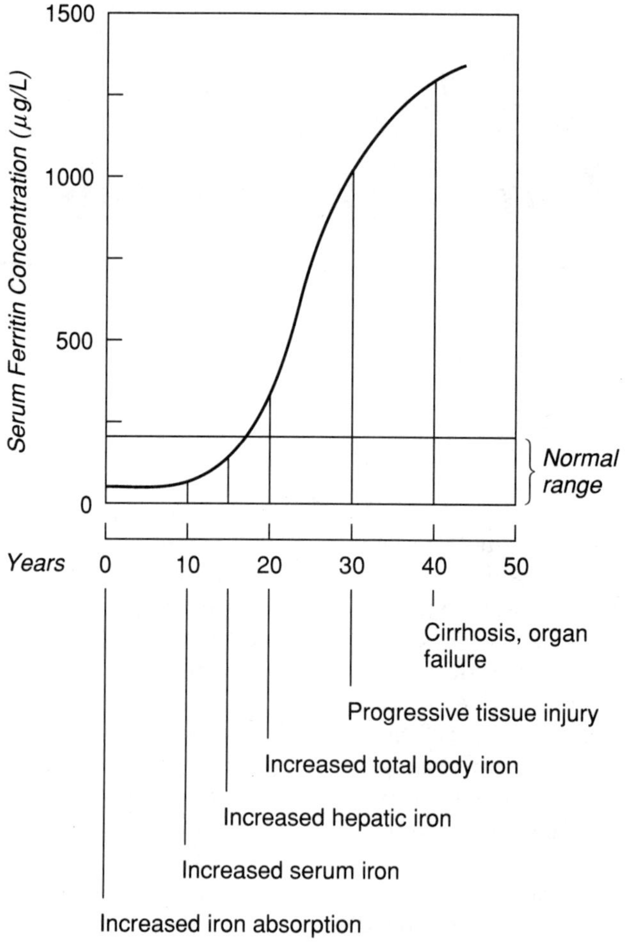

Fig. 14-1. The sequence of events in inherited hemochromatosis and their correlation with iron overload, as measured by the serum ferritin (1 μg/L of ferritin corresponds to 7.5 mg of body iron in the absence of liver disease or inflammation). If untreated, iron overload will result in a decrease of life expectancy, with hepatocellular carcinoma being the most common cause of death, followed by heart failure, cirrhosis, and diabetes. (From Powell LW, Isselbacher KJ: Hemochromatosis. In Wilson JD et al. (eds.): Harrison's Principles of Internal Medicine, 12 Ed. McGraw-Hill, New York, 1991, with permission.)

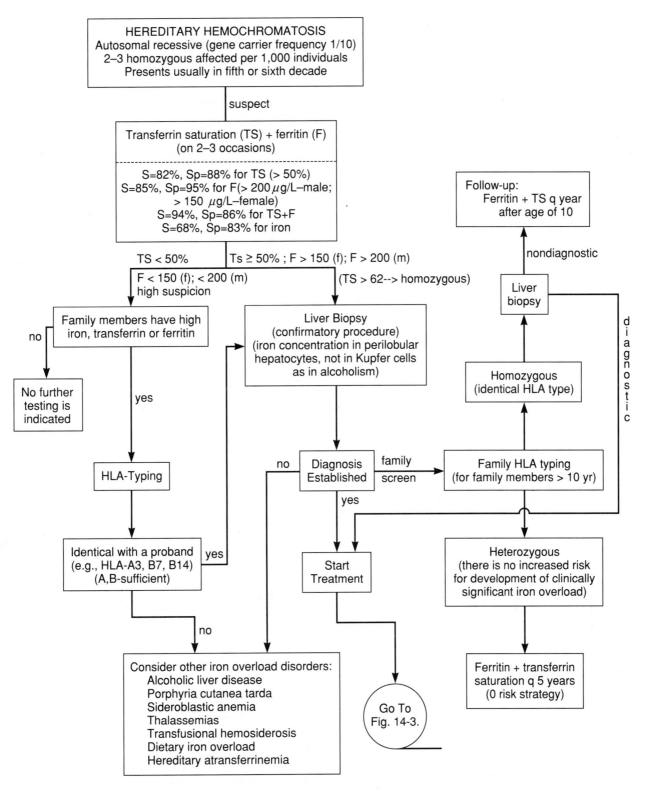

Fig. 14-2. An algorithm for the diagnosis of hemochromatosis. The *probabilistic approach* is applied to the construction of this algorithm, which is based upon the application of tests with the highest predictive values (TS + F) in the setting of the disease with a high prevalence (see also Fig. 1-4). Note that screening is recommended in the setting of a high pretest probability of disease (family, certain ethnic groups).

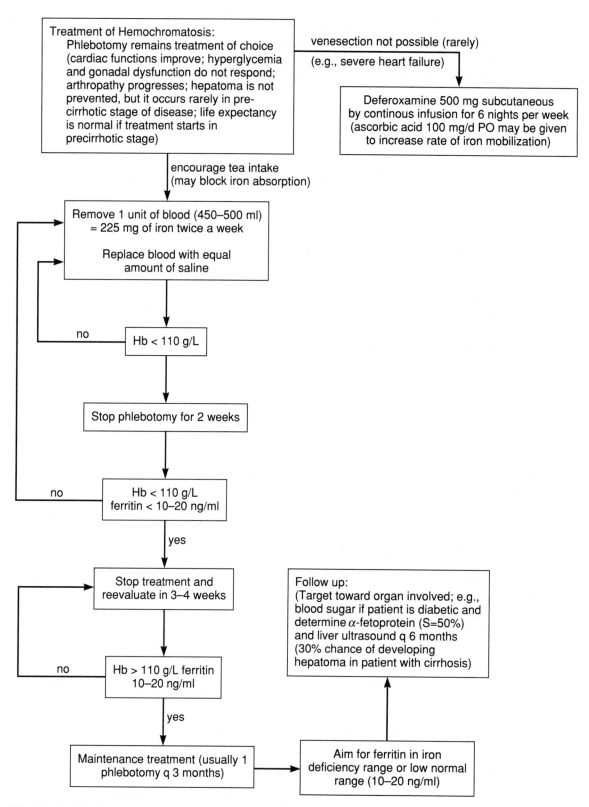

Fig. 14-3. An algorithm for the treatment of hemochromatosis. It is constructed upon the understanding of the pathophysiology of disease (i.e., there is a cause-effect relationship between iron overload and organ damage) (see Fig. 14-1). The logical approach is to decrease the iron burden in the patient and monitor the degree of that burden (*a causal model of clinical reasoning*).

(or iron chelation if venesection is not possible). Figure 14-3 shows an algorithm for the *treatment* of hemochromatosis. Life expectancy of these patients approaches normal if treatment starts early. The development of hepatoma is, however, not prevented if treatment starts when patients have already developed cirrhosis. Note that heterozygotes do have a normal life expectancy.

Suggested Readings

Adams PC, Halliday JW, Powell LW: Early diagnosis and treatment of hemochromatosis. Adv Intern Med 34:111, 1989

Adams PC, Kertesz AE, Valberg LS: Clinical presentation of hemochromatosis: a changing scene. Am J Med 90:445, 1991

Bassett ML, Halliday JW, Ferris RA, Powell LW: Diagnosis of hemochromatosis in young subjects: predictive accuracy of biochemical screening tests. Gastroenterology 87:628, 1989

Holland HK, Spivak JL: Hemochromatosis. Med Clin North Am 73:831, 1989

Niederau C: Survival and cause of death in cirrhotic and in noncirrhotic patients with primary hemochromatosis. N Engl J Med 313:1256, 1985

Ulvik RJ: Screening for hemochromatosis. Scand J Clin Lab Med 90, 1990

15 | Porphyrias: Diagnosis

Porphyrias are inborn errors in heme production, and are labeled as *erythropoietic* (congenital erythropoietic porphyria—CEP), *hepatic* (acute intermittent porphyria—AIP; porphyria cutanea tarda—PCT; hereditary coproporphyria—HC; variegate porphyria—PV), or *erythrohepatic* (protoporphyria—PP), depending on whether the enzyme deficiency appears in the red blood cells (RBCs), the liver, or both. The prevalence for these disorders is estimated to range between 3.4–7.7 per 100,000 people (AIP and PV) to extremely rare diseases such as CEP (less than 200 cases reported). In North America, AIP and PCT are the two most common forms of porphyria, with an AIP prevalence of 210 per 100,000 in the psychiatric population and PCT being more frequent in the alcoholic population. With the exception of CEP, which is inherited through an autosomal recessive pattern, all other porphyrias are inherited in the autosomal dominant fashion. The diagnosis is usually made in the second or third decade of life in cases of hepatic porphyrias, with the exception of PCT, which is usually diagnosed between the ages of 40–60; cases of erythropoietic and erythrohepatic porphyrias are usually diagnosed in childhood.

The clinical picture can be derived from the nature of the biochemical effect: if *porphyrin precursors* (δ-aminolevulinic acid—ALA, porphobilinogen—PBG) are overproduced, a patient will have *gastrointestinal and neuropsychiatric manifestations* (these symptoms vary from typical abdominal pain to ileus, and from depression to respiratory failure or coma); if *porphyrins* are overproduced, the main manifestation will be *skin lesions*. Thus, AIP does *not* show

skin lesions, and HC will uncommonly manifest with skin lesions. On the other hand, PCT and PP do *not* go with abdominal pain.

In patients presenting with abdominal pain (and overproduction of porphyrin precursors such as ALA and PBG), only three differential diagnostic possibilities exist: AIP, HC, and PV. Positive skin lesions essentially excludes AIP, but negative is of no help. Biochemical determination of porphyrins and their precursors in urine, feces, and most recently in bile, will help make this distinction. It should be noted that PBG and ALA are *always* (S = 100%) increased in urine in AIP, irrespective of the clinical picture (acute attack *vs* asymptomatic; normal result excludes AIP). This, however, is not the case in HC and PV, which usually have negative tests when they are not acutely ill. In these cases, porphyrin analysis in the stool or bile will be of help (Fig. 15-1).

"Screening tests" for porphyrias based upon qualitative determination of PBG in the urine using the Watson-Schwartz or the Hoesch test have poor sensitivity (40–69% when the urine sample is dark-colored and 28–53% when the urine is normal-colored), and cannot be used for this purpose. These tests should be considered obsolete and replaced by quantitative determination of PBG and ALA. Significant increases in urinary PBG and ALA makes the diagnosis of AIP, VP, or HCP highly likely (specificity near 100%), and a normal result of a quantitative test for urine PBG makes the diagnosis of porphyria in patients with acute symptoms highly unlikely (sensitivity near 100%). Still, the Watson-Schwartz test is almost always positive during episodes of neu-

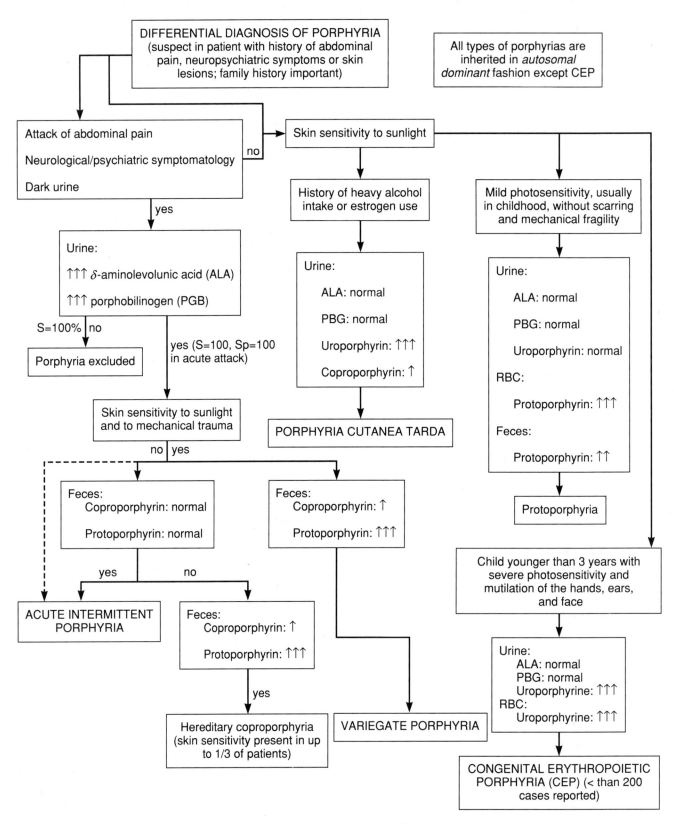

Fig. 15-1. Algorithm for differential diagnosis of porphyria. Physiologic reasoning directs the first step in differential diagnosis: skin *vs* gastrointestinal/neuropsychiatric manifestations. Further distinction is based upon a combination of *probabilistic* (prevalence of skin lesions, increase in metabolites of interest—i.e., test positivity depending upon acute attack of disease) and *physiologic* reasoning (measuring of metabolite of interest depending on the enzyme defect involved). Note that detection of the level of enzymes, such as porphobilinogen deaminase (the enzyme affected in AIP), is not included in the algorithm, because these levels cannot discriminate between carriers and affected individuals.

Table 15-1. Operating Characteristics of Tests Used in Diagnosis of Porphyria

Test	Sensitivity (%)	Specificity (%)	Disease
Urinary ALA and PBG increase	100	?	AIP (no symptoms)
Urinary ALA and PBG increase	100	100	AIP, VP, HC (with symptoms)
RBC porphobilinogen deaminase	90	98	AIP
Watson-Schwartz test	40–60	?	AIP
Dark urine	74	?	AIP, VP, HC
Abdominal pain	95	?	AIP (hospital admission)
Peripheral motor deficit	60	?	AIP

ropsychiatric dysfunction, and a positive result is probably justification for intravenous administration of glucose while waiting for the results of a quantitative analysis. Operating characteristics of tests used in diagnosis of porphyria are shown in Table 15-1.

Suggested Readings

Bonkovsky HL: Porphyria: Practical advice for the clinical gastroenterologist and hepatologist. Dig Dis 179:5, 1987

Buttery JE, Carrera AM, Pannall PR: Reliability of the porphobilinogen screening assay. Pathology 22:197, 1990

Deacon AC: Performance of screening tests for porphyria. Ann Clin Biochem 25:392, 1988

Kushner JP: Laboratory diagnosis of the porphyrias. N Engl J Med 324:1432, 1991

Pierach CA, Weimer MK, Cardinal RA, et al.: Red blood cell porphobilinogen deaminase in the evaluation of acute intermittent porphyria. JAMA 257:60, 1987

Schreiber WE, Jamani A, Pudek MR: Screening tests for porphobilinogen are insensitive. The problem and its solution. Am J Clin Pathol 92:644, 1989

16 | Porphyrias: Treatment

Three hepatic porphyrias—*acute intermittent porphyria* (AIP), *hereditary coproporphyria* (HC), and *variegate porphyria* (VP)—are known as *"acute attack"* porphyrias because they have two major clinical manifestations in common: attacks of abdominal pain and neuropsychiatric symptoms. Principles of treatment involve preventive management and treatment of acute attacks, the latter involving symptomatic measures and physiologic targeting of the rate-limiting enzyme δ-aminolevulinic acid (ALA) synthetase. During acute attacks, the differentiation between AIP, HC, and VP is of little practical importance, since treatment is the same for all.

Immediate withdrawal of all possible offending drugs is the first logical step in the therapeutic approach to the patient with AIP, HC, or VP. Some common drugs that are known to precipitate porphyric attacks, as well as some considered to be safe, are shown in Figure 16-1. It is rational to avoid the use of drugs whose effect on acute hepatic porphyrias is unknown.

The treatment of an acute attack includes the administration of carbohydrate, and/or hematin, correction of electrolyte abnormalities, and general supportive care. Chlorpromazine may be useful in treating abdominal pain, presumably in part through its ganglionic blocking activity, but for some patients narcotic analgesics (morphine, meperidine, or codeine) are necessary. Monitoring of electrolytes is essential to prevent or correct hyponatremia, hypomagnesemia, and eventually hypokalemia, which may be present during the administration of glucose.

A high-carbohydrate intake is aimed at suppression of the rate-limiting enzyme ALA synthetase. A carbohydrate is given as an intravenous 10% dextrose solution in amounts approaching 500 grams per day. The response to carbohydrate intake is variable; some patients show obvious improvement, whereas others are not affected. By carefully monitoring urinary excretion of PBG, it is possible to predict the course of an acute attack: a decrease in urinary PBG may herald clinical improvement, while a rise in urinary PBG may be followed by the progression of neurologic manifestations and respiratory failure. It is therefore useful to measure urinary excretion of PBG (and ALA) every day during an acute attack, when it can range from 50–200 mg/day (normal urinary PBG is less than 2 mg/24 hours). There is current evidence that hematin (a hydroxide of hemoglobin) is more effective than glucose in reducing this excretion; therefore, in patients with significant neurologic symptoms or in those who fail to respond to glucose (see algorithm), hematin is given. Hematin therapy is clinically effective in over 90% of patients.

During the course of an acute attack, structural changes in the neuronal tissues may occur that are irreversible (or require a *long* time to heal). It is therefore important (especially in patients with significant neurologic involvement) to give hematin early in the course of the disease, when structural changes have not yet occurred. A clinical response to hematin may not be observed for at least 48 hours, and usually occurs on the third or fourth day of treatment. The decrease in urinary PBG generally pre-

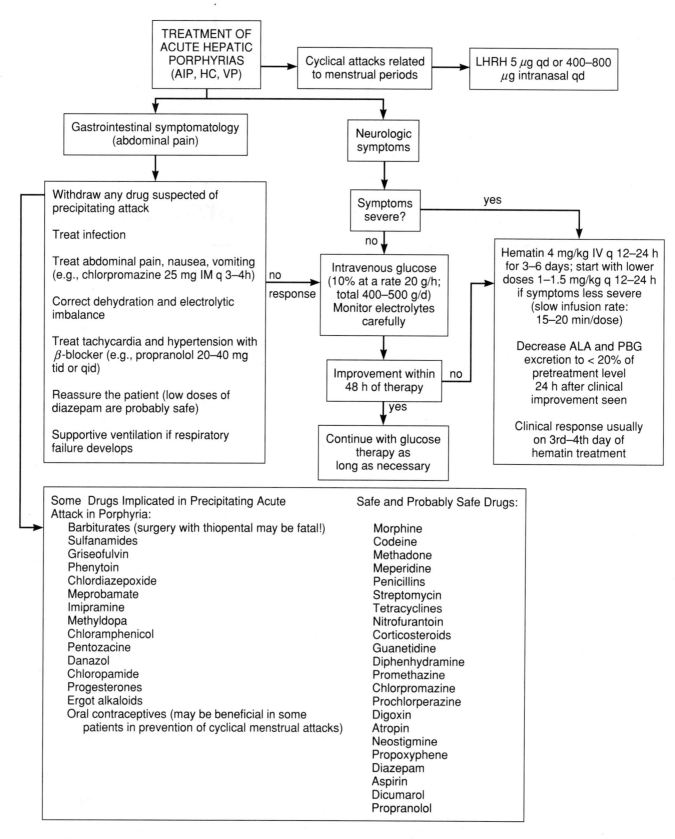

Fig. 16-1. Management of acute hepatic porphyrias. Prevention and treatment of acute attacks are the two principles involved. Treatment is based upon *physiologic* line of reasoning and includes symptomatic therapy and targeting of the rate-limiting enzyme (ALA synthetase), thought to be responsible for over-production of porphyrin precursors, which in turn cause clinical manifestations.

cedes the clinical response by 24 hours. Solutions of lyophilized hematin are reconstituted immediately before infusion, because freshly prepared hematin does not affect coagulation, while a decayed solution does (prolongation of prothrombin and thromboplastin times, a decrease in fibrinogen, thrombocytopenia).

The preventive approach involves the avoidance of precipitating factors as mentioned above, and in cases of *cyclical attack* of AIP, administration of long-acting agonists of luteinizing hormone-releasing hormone. This therapy, however, still needs future clinical trials to elucidate its real role in the treatment of porphyria.

Suggested Readings

Anderson KE: LHRH analogues for hormonal manipulation in acute intermittent porphyria. Semin Hematol 26:10, 1989

Billett HH: Porphyrias: Inborn errors in heme production. Hosp Pract September 30:41, 1988

Herrick AL, McColl KE, Moore MR, Cook A, Goldberg A: A controlled trial of haem arginate in acute hepatic porphyria. Lancet i:1295, 1989

Ippen H, Fuchs T: What is guaranteed in therapy of acute intermittent porphyria. Internist 31:698, 1990

Mustajaki P, Tenhunen R, Pierach C, Volin L: Heme in the treatment of porphyrias and hematologic disorders. Semin Hematol 26:1, 1989

17 | Hyperbilirubinemia

Occasionally, hematologists will be asked to consult on a patient presenting with increased bilirubin. Clinical workup in this case is based upon a combination of physiologic and probabilistic reasoning. The first question is whether the jaundice is due to predominantly unconjugated hyperbilirubinemia or conjugated hyperbilirubinemia. *Unconjugated hyperbilirubinemia* can reflect hematologic pathology or liver pathology. There are only two hematologic conditions that can produce unconjugated hyperbilirubinemia: *hemolysis* and *ineffective erythropoiesis*. Hemolytic anemia (HA) is the most common cause of unconjugated hyperbilirubinemia, and the reticulocyte count is the single most useful test in the initial workup of patients with HA (see Chapters 3 and 8). The second most common cause of unconjugated hyperbilirubinemia is Gilbert syndrome.

In the approach to the patient presenting with *conjugated hyperbilirubinemia*, the key question is distinguishing between *medical* (hepatocellular) and *surgical* (biliary obstruction) causes of jaundice. The choice of diagnostic tests will depend on their operating characteristics (see Table 17-1). Ultrasound (US) is usually the initial procedure of choice because of its high accuracy in demonstrating the presence or absence of dilated bile ducts. Some authors prefer a computerized tomography (CT) because of slightly better operating characteristics, but this test carries a risk of irradiation and is more expensive. Percutaneous transhepatic cholangiography (PTC) and endoscopic retrograde cholangiopancreatography (ERCP) are highly sensitive and specific tests for the obstruction site. A negative US and CT virtually exclude extrahepatic obstructive disease, in which case consideration should be given to a liver biopsy. It is important to stress that the most common disorders associated with jaundice are hepatitis and cirrhosis, and that the most common causes of ductal obstruction are choledocholithiasis and malignancy.

A combination of test operating characteristics with pretest estimates of the existence of a particular disease can give a precise calculation of the probability of obstructive or hepatocellular jaundice (see Chapter 1). Figure 17.1. shows an algorithm for the clinical workup of hyperbilirubinemia.

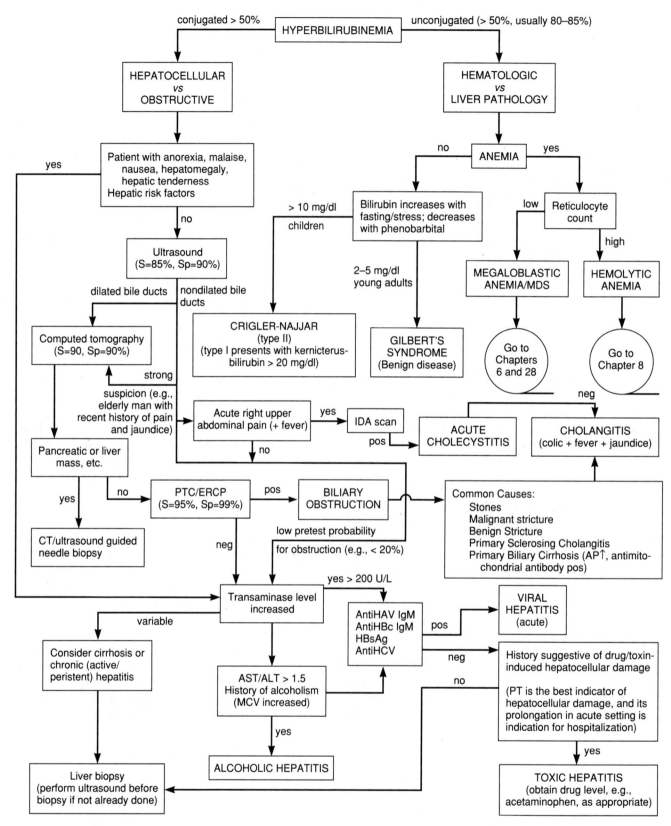

Fig. 17-1. An algorithm for clinical workup of hyperbilirubinemia. It starts with *physiologic* principles (conjugated *vs* unconjugated, hematologic *vs* liver pathology, hepatocellular *vs* obstructive jaundice). Further workup is *probabilistic,* based upon operating test characteristics of the diagnostic tests. Note that rare causes of conjugated hyperbilirubinemia, such as Rotor and Dubin-Johnson syndrome, are not shown.

Table 17-1. Operating Characteristics of Diagnostic Tests Used in Evaluation of Patients With Hyperbilirubinemia

Diagnostic Test	Sensitivity (%)	Specificity (%)	Disease
History and physical exam and routine laboratory tests	95	76	Extrahepatic obstruction
Abdominal pain	70	68	Extrahepatic obstruction
US	85	90–95	Extrahepatic obstruction
CT	90	90–95	Extrahepatic obstruction
ERCP/PTC	95	99	Extrahepatic obstruction
Alkaline phosphatase (AP) (>3 times normal)	85	65	Extrahepatic obstruction
AST/ALT > 1.5 + MCV > 90	97	89	Alcoholic hepatitis
AST (units/L):			
200–400	73	98	Viral hepatitis
401–600	57	99	Viral hepatitis
>600	50	>99	Viral hepatitis
IgM anti-HAV	99	99	Hepatitis A
IgM anti-HBc	90	98	Hepatitis B
HBsAg	80	97	Hepatitis B
Anti-HCV	87	89	Hepatitis C

Symptoms	Pretest Probabilities (%)	Disease/Condition
Malaise, anorexia, nausea	90	Acute hepatitis
Adult with abdominal pain	60	Obstructive jaundice
Adult (>40)	40	Obstructive jaundice
Palpable gallbladder	100	Obstructive jaundice
Hemophiliac	10	Hepatitis B
Spouse or sexual partner of hepatitis B patient	25	Hepatitis B

[a] Use this table with the nomogram in Fig. 1-6 to calculate post-test probabilities.

Suggested Readings

Arvan DA: Obstructive jaundice. In Panzer RJ, Black E, Griner PF (eds.): Diagnostic strategies for common medical problems. American College of Physicians, Philadelphia, 131, 1990

Fevery J, Blanckaert N: What can we learn from analysis of serum bilirubin? Hepatol 2:113, 1986

Frank BB: Clinical evaluation of jaundice. JAMA 262:3031, 1989

Kawachi I, Robinson GM, Stace NH: A combination of raised serum AST:ALT ratio and erythrocyte mean cell volume level detects excessive alcohol consumption. N Z Med J 103:145, 1990

Khoo US, Lavelle SM: The utility of ancillary tests in diagnosis of jaundice. Med Inf (Lond) 13:93, 1988

Lindsell DR: Ultrasound imaging of pancreas and biliary tract. Lancet 335:390, 1990

Olsson R, Stigendal L: Clinical experience with isolated hyperbilirubinemia. Scand J Gastroenterol 24:617, 1989

Scharschmidt BF, Goldbery HI, Schmid R: Approach to the patient with cholestatic jaundice. N Engl J Med 308:1515, 1983

18 | Diagnostic Approach to Polycythemia

An elevated hemoglobin and hematocrit can occur due to an *absolute* erythrocytosis (elevated red cell mass) or *relative* erythrocytosis (reduced plasma volume). An absolute erythrocytosis can occur due to *polycythemia rubra vera*—P. Vera (a clonal myeloproliferative disorder) or to disorders associated with elevated erythropoietin (secondary erythrocytosis). Figure 18-1 shows the physiologic approach to the differential diagnosis of polycythemia. Although the best way to distinguish absolute from relative erythrocytosis is by Cr^{51} isotope studies, there is a direct relationship between the level of the hematocrit and the probability that the red cell mass is truly increased (Fig. 18-2). It can be noted that for a hematocrit >60% in males and >55% in females, there is a 99% probability that the red cell mass is truly increased. In these circumstances, one does not have to order radioisotope studies to find out whether the high hematocrit is due to reasons of absolute or relative erythrocytosis. A diagnosis of the specific entity causing polycythemia will depend on the prevalence of disease(s) (pretest probability) that may cause polycythemia, test operating characteristics (i.e., its sensitivity and specificity), and test availability to the physician (availability heuristic).

The first box below shows the prevalence of the most common causes of polycythemia, with the most common by far being smoking. In the nonsmokers' group, P. Vera is the most probable etiological reason for a high hematocrit. The second box shows the criteria of the Polycythemia Vera Study Group for diagnosis of P. Rubra Vera. While helpful, these criteria are quite rigid. At a low pretest probability (such as in the case of young smokers), one should have the Polycythemia Vera Study Group criteria fulfilled in order to establish a diagnosis of P. Vera. At high pretest probabilities (older patients, nonsmokers), this would not be necessary, and fulfillment of only two major criteria would sometimes be enough (Fig. 18-3). One has to stress that splenomegaly is the most important finding for a diagnosis of P. Vera. In patients with a high hematocrit, splenomegaly is almost 100% specific for P. Vera (see second box). The operative test characteristics of other useful tests in the workup of polycythemia are shown in Table 18-1. An algorithm for the diagnosis

---

Prevalance of the Most Common Causes of Polycythemia

Smoking: 600–1,000/100,000
P. Vera: 10/100,000
Tumors: .2–.7/100,000

Probability of the Etiology of Polycythemia

Smokers:	Nonsmokers:
Smoking (98%)	P. Vera (33%)
P. Vera (1%)	Relative
Tumors and other	erythrocytosis
causes (1%)	(65%)
	Tumors and other
	causes (1%)

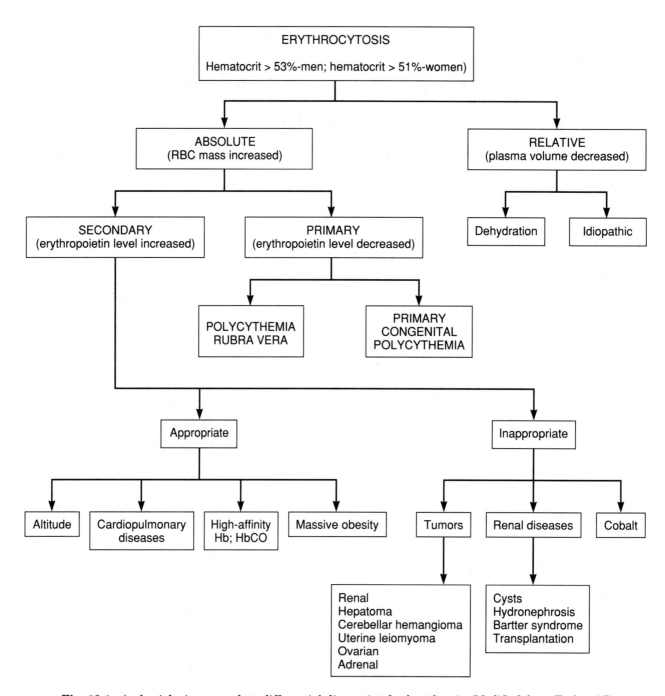

Fig. 18-1. A physiologic approach to differential diagnosis of polycythemia (Modified from Erslev AD: Primary and secondary erythrocytosis. In Brain MC, Carbone PP (eds): Current Therapy in Hematology-Oncology-3. BC Decker, Toronto, 1988.)

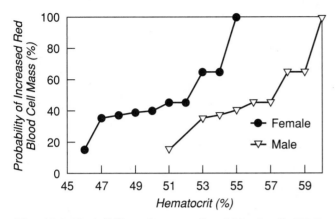

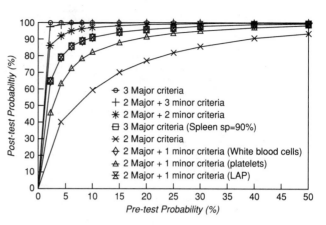

Fig. 18-2. Probability of increased red blood cell (RBC) mass as a function of hematocrit. For a hematocrit > 60% in men or > 55% in women, there is a 99% probability that the patient has an absolute increase in RBC mass. (From Djulbegovic et al.: Am Fam Physician 44:113, 1991, with permission.)

Fig. 18-3. Evaluation of the predictive value of the Polycythemia Vera Study Group criteria for the diagnosis of P. vera. The requirement of three minor criteria may be appropriate to make the diagnosis in the absence of splenomegaly if there is a low probability for P. Vera (e.g., young patients, smokers, patients with COPD, etc.). On the other hand, in the high pretest probability setting (e.g., 55-year-old nonsmoker without history of COPD), it may be justifiable to make a diagnosis of P. Vera based upon two major criteria only. Note that treatment thresholds may be as low as 32% (see Chapter 19). (From Djulbegovic et al.: Am Fam Physician 44:113, 1991, with permission.)

Polycythemia Vera Study Group Criteria for Diagnosis of
Polycythemia Rubra Vera: Production Rule No. 1

Category A
A1: Total RBC volume:
Male ≥36 ml/kg of body weight
Female ≥32 ml/kg of body weight
A2: Arterial saturation O_2 > 92%
A3: Splenomegaly

Category B
B1: Thrombocytosis >400,000/mm³
B2: Leukocytosis >12,000/mm³ (no fever or infection)
B3: Leukocyte alkaline phosphatase (LAP) core score > 100
B4: Serum vitamin B_{12} (>900 pg/ml) or $UB_{12}BC$ (>2,200 pg/ml)

Polycythemia Vera: A1 + A2 + A3
or
A1 + A2 + any two from category B

(Note that criteria are, in fact, production rules derived from the understanding of the pathophysiology of the process and clinical picture of the disease. Data from Berlin: Semin Hematol 12:339, 1975)

Polycythemia Rubra Vera: Production Rule No. 2

If patient has an increased hematocrit <u>and</u> splenomegaly, *then* suspect P. Vera until proven otherwise.

(Note that this production rule was derived from a statistical association of splenomegaly with a high hematocrit.)

Polycythemia: Production Rule No. 3

If patient has family history positive for increased RBC count, *then* suspect high affinity hemoglobin or primary congenital polycythemia.

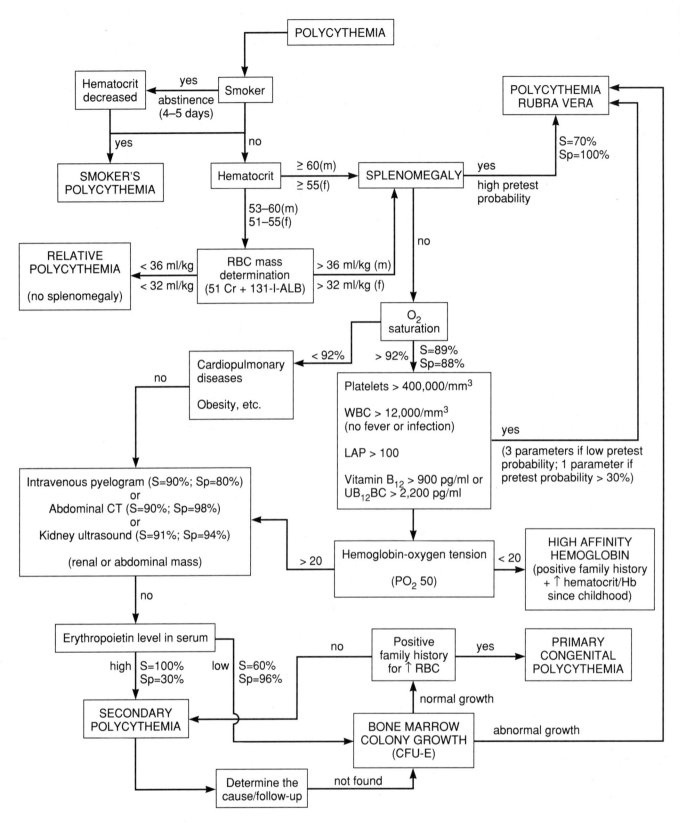

Fig. 18-4. An algorithm for diagnosis of polycythemia. The optimal approach involves a combination of *probabilistic, deterministic,* and *causal* reasoning, plus an availability of data that will trigger certain diagnostic hypotheses (principle of availability heuristic) (e.g., a hematocrit >60% in 60-year-old non-smoker will immediately trigger a hypothesis of P. Vera, i.e., search for splenomegaly). (From Djulbegovic et al.: Am Fam Physician 44:113, 1991, with permission.)

Table 18-1. Operating Test Characteristics of Diagnostic Tests Used in Work-up of Patients With Elevated Hematocrit

Test	Sensitivity (%)	Specificity (%)	Disease
Age (>40)	95	2–33	PRV
Smoking	5	98	SmP
RBC mass (Cr method)	90	50	PRV
O_2 saturation (> 92%)	89	88	PRV
Splenomegaly	70	100	PRV
WBC (>12,000)	43	94	PRV
Platelets (>400,000)	63	80	PRV
LAP score (>100)	70	90	PRV
B_{12} level	36	70	PRV
$UB_{12}BC$	98	87	PRV
P. Vera Criteria	65–70	80–85	PRV
CFU-E	93–100	100	PRV
Serum Epo (low level)	31–94	92–100	PRV
Serum Epo (high level)	67–100	13–31	SP
IVP	90	80	RT
Abdominal CT	90–100	98	RT
Ultrasound	84–98	88–100	RC

Abbreviations: PVR, Polycythemia rubra vera; SmP, smoker's polycythemia; SP, secondary polycythemia; RT, renal tumor; RC, renal cyst; CFU-E RBC, progenitor cells (performed without adding erythropoietin (Epo) to in vitro culture system, as is usually done). (From Djulbegovic et al: Am Fam Physician 44:113, 1991, with permission.)

of polycythemia is shown in Figure 18-4. Note that *positive family history* regarding increased red blood cell (RBC) count can trigger two hypotheses—high affinity hemoglobin, and/or primary congenital polycythemia. However, even in this (younger) group of patients, other causes of polycythemia (e.g., kidney diseases) will be more frequent and should be excluded first. Similarly, determination of pO_2-50% and bone marrow colony growth are still not widely available tests, making the strategy presented in Figure 18-4 the most cost-effective.

Suggested Readings

Baclerzak SP, Bromberg PA: Secondary polycythemia. Semin Hematol 12:353, 1975

Berlin NI: Diagnosis and classification of polycythemias. Semin Hematol 12:339, 1975

Budd JL, Greenland P: Erythrocytosis. In Griner P, Panzer RJ, Greenland P (eds.): Clinical Diagnosis and Laboratory: Logical Strategies to Common Medical Problems. Year Book, Chicago, 1986

Djulbegovic B, Hadley T, Joseph G: A new algorithm for diagnosis of polycythemia. Am Fam Physician 44:113, 1991

Smith JR, Landow SA: Smokers polycythemia. N Engl J Med 298:6, 1978

Treatment of Polycythemia Rubra Vera (PRV) and Secondary Polycythemia

19

Should PRV be treated? Left untreated, patients with PRV do poorly, and 50% die within 18 months of the onset of the first sign or symptom. With therapy, a dramatic improvement in survival has been reported, with a median survival of 8–15 years. The leading causes of mortality in PRV are hemorrhagic and thrombotic complications in cerebral, coronary, and pulmonary circulatory systems.

Who should be treated? Using the threshold concept shown in Chapter 1, it can be calculated that (depending on the type of treatment and its accompanying risks) treatment may be indicated if the probability that the patient has PRV exceeds 32% (treatment thresholds range: 10–62%) (see also Fig. 18-3). Every PRV patient with an increased hematocrit and/or thrombotic complications should be treated; the cerebral blood flow decreases when the hematocrit is above 53%, and cerebral function is improved by reduction of the hematocrit below 45%.

How should PRV be treated? Therapy should be individualized according to the patient's age and severity of disease. Generally, the induction regimen should consist of phlebotomy, with maintenance adjusted according to the patient's age: patients younger than 50 should be treated with phlebotomy alone; patients between 50–70 years of age should be treated with phlebotomy and/or myelosuppression; and older patients are probably best treated with ^{32}P. The choice of therapy is based on the number of complications involved in these long-term treatments, the probability of adequate control of the disease, and compliance with treatment. Thus, phlebotomy is preferred in young patients because of the low frequency of side effects. However, phlebotomy does not control thrombocytosis, leukocytosis, painful spleen, and other manifestations of the disease, and, therefore, myelosuppression is the choice of treatment in the older group of patients. (Thrombosis is the cause of 47% of deaths in patients treated with phlebotomy alone and 28–31% of patients treated with myelosuppression and radioactive phosphor, respectively). The *therapeutic dilemma* is reflected in the choice of phlebotomy, with an unacceptable high incidence of thrombotic events (the major risk factors for thrombosis are phlebotomy, history of previous thrombosis, and advanced age), and myelosuppressive therapy, with the risk of development of secondary malignancies. Figures 19-1 (A, B, and C) show recommended treatment approaches to P. Vera. It should also be mentioned that antiplatelet agents (aspirin + dipyridamole) do not reduce the frequency of thrombotic events; in fact, their use has been associated with an increased incidence of gastrointestinal hemorrhages. Recently, however, preliminary data has shown that the use of ticlopidine reduces the risk of thrombosis. Another treatment dilemma is the treatment of iron deficiency in PRV patients: if iron is given, it can stimulate production of RBC; if it is withdrawn, severe microcytosis can occur, which increases blood viscosity even further. One recommended compromise is to administer iron when mean cell hemoglobin concentration (MCHC) is less than 22 pg, with careful monitoring of Hb and hematocrit.

How should therapy be monitored? The goal of therapy should be to retain the hematocrit in a range between 42–47% and the number of platelets below 600×10^9L. These recommendations do not relate

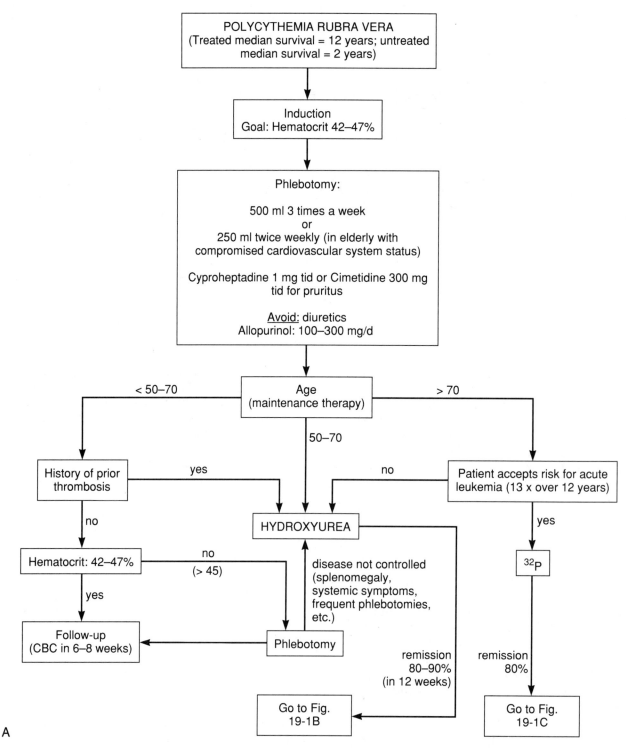

Fig. 19-1 (A, B, and C). An algorithm for the treatment of P. Vera. Initiation of therapy is *threshold driven* (see text), but is based upon the understanding of the *physiologic consequences* of the high hematocrit for microvascular circulation. The choice of therapy depends on the *risk/benefit* considerations of the effectiveness of the treatment and its adverse effects. ^{32}P is the most convenient (and probably the most effective), but also the riskiest therapy. Phlebotomy, history of previous thrombosis, and advanced age are the major risks for thrombosis (leading cause of death). Mutagenic potential of hydroxyurea is still not fully evaluated at this time. α-interferon is reserved as a last treatment of choice because, at this time, its role is not fully evaluated.

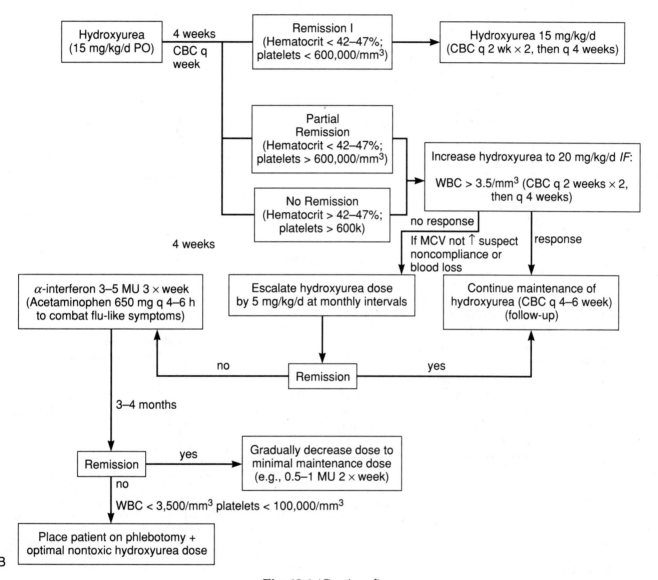

Fig. 19-1 (*Continued*)

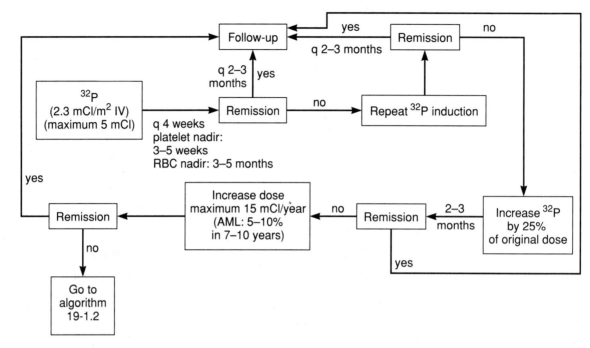

Fig. 19-1 (*Continued*)

to *primary congenital polycythemia*, a disorder usually inherited in autosomal dominant fashion, which is an essentially benign condition and usually does not require treatment.

In *secondary polycythemia* due to COPD *or* cyanotic heart disease, the hematocrit should be maintained at about 50% and between 55–60%, respectively. Although it does not seem that high-affinity hemoglobins reduce survival, the majority of authors recommend keeping the hematocrit between 55–60%. It should also be stressed that *surgical mortality* is increased in patients with PRV. The risk is reduced after the disease has been controlled for approximately 4 months.

Suggested Readings

Berk PD, Goldberg JD, Donovan PB, et al.: Therapeutic recommendations in polycythemia vera based upon Polycythemia Vera Study Group protocols. Semin Hematol 23:132, 1986

Erslev AD: Primary and secondary erythrocytosis. In Brain MC, Carbone PP (eds.): Current therapy in hematology-oncology-3. B.C. Decker, Toronto/Philadelphia, 1988

Fruchtman SM, Wasserman LR, Berk PD: Polycythemia rubra vera. In Brain MC, Carbone PP (eds.): Current therapy in hematology-oncology-3. B.C. Decker, Toronto/Philadelphia, 1988

Kaplan ME, Mack K, Goldberg JD, et al.: Long-term management of polycythemia vera with hydroxyurea: a progress report. Semin Hematol 23:167, 1986

Prchal JT, Crist WM, Goldwasser E, et al.: Autosomal dominant polycythemia. Blood 66:1208, 1985

Silver RT: A new treatment for polycythemia vera: recombinant interferon alfa. Blood 76:664, 1990

Tartaglia AP, Goldberg JD, Berk PD, Wasserman LR: Adverse effects of anti-aggregating platelet therapy in the treatment of polycythemia vera. Semin Hematol 23:172, 1986

20 | Methemoglobinemia

Methemoglobinemia refers to the condition in which more than 1% of the hemoglobin (Hb) of the blood has been oxidized to the ferric form. This condition may be *hereditary* or *acquired*. Genetic defects in the structure of the globin molecule (Hb M) or a deficiency of the enzyme cytochrome b_5 reductase (NADH-diaphorase) are the two most common causes of hereditary methemoglobinemia. In the so-called type II NADH-diaphorase deficiency, progressive encephalopathy and mental retardation are commonly found. Hb M disease is an autosomal dominant disorder, and the NADH-diaphorase condition is autosomal recessively inherited. Acquired methemoglobinemia occurs when various drugs or toxic substances oxidize Hb directly or help its oxidation by molecular oxygen. Nitrites, aniline derivatives, and sulfonamides are the most common culprits.

A *production rule* derived from knowledge of the prevalence of conditions causing *cyanosis* may be of help in diagnosing methemoglobinemia: *If* a patient presenting with a cyanosis has intact cardiovascular and respiratory systems, *then* suspect methemoglobinemia. As little as 1.5 g/dl of methemoglobin is sufficient to produce cyanosis. (Also, cyanosis can occur when the concentration of reduced hemoglobin exceeds 5 g/dl, or when there is more than 0.5 g/dl of sulfhemoglobin. Cyanosis due to high-affinity hemoglobin is due to a compensatory increase in red blood cell (RBC) mass.) A diagnosis of methemoglobinemia should be suspected when blood appears chocolate-brown in color. NADH-diaphorase activity is low if this enzyme-deficiency condition exists. Hb M can be differentiated from methemoglobin spectroscopically or by electrophoresis if the former is suspected. A key diagnostic finding in methemoglobinemia is normal pO_2 (blood count is typically normal, although mild polycythemia may occasionally be found).

There is a correlation between levels of methemoglobin and symptoms with levels >50% being potentially fatal. This is especially true in acquired (toxic) methemoglobinemia when symptoms develop rapidly. Prompt institution of therapy is of utmost importance in these cases (see Fig. 20-1 for details of management). In general, the prognosis in hereditary types of methemoglobinemia is good, and these types usually present no problems outside of cosmetic concerns. Patients, however, should avoid exposure to drugs known to induce methemoglobinemia. The same relates to *sulfhemoglobinemia*, which is an essentially benign disorder.

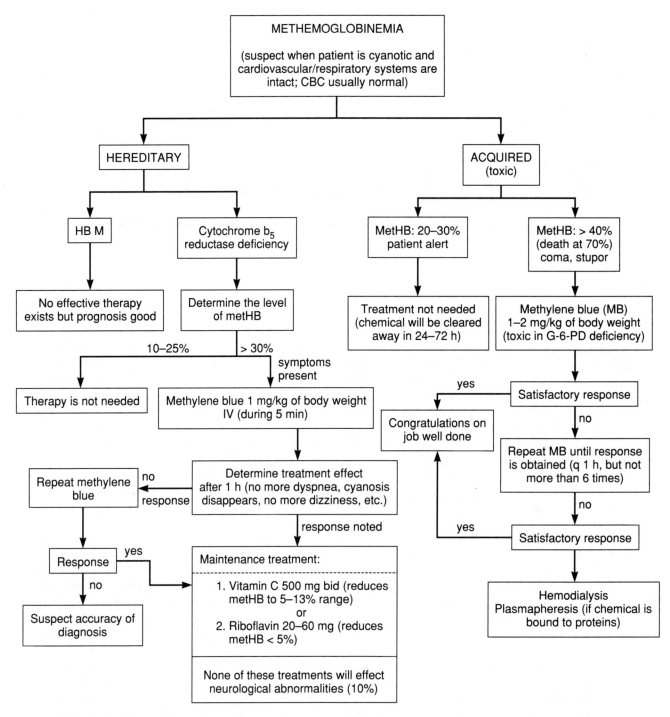

Fig. 20-1. Physiologic (*causal*) approach to the treatment of methemoglobinemia. Treatment is based upon an understanding of the biochemical defects of the alteration of hem(oglobin) molecule and its physiologic consequences. Figure relates to G-6-PD nondeficient individuals. Note that MB is contraindicated in G-6-PD deficient individuals. In these cases, RBC transfusion, oxygen, and/or exchange transfusion may be needed.

Suggested Readings

Hegesh E, Hegesh J, Kaftory A: Congenital methemoglobinemia with a deficiency of cytochrome b_5. N Engl J Med 314:757, 1986

Lukens JN: The legacy of well-water methemoglobinemia. JAMA 257:2793, 1987

Park CM, Nagel RL: Sulfhemoglobinemia. Clinical and molecular aspects. N Engl J Med 310:1579, 1984

21 | Leukocytosis

Leukocytosis is usually defined as occurring when the total white blood cell (WBC) count exceeds 10,000/mm³ (10 × 10⁹/L). (Interestingly, there is considerable disagreement on just what a normal count is; see Table 21-1 for a summary of the studies on normal complete blood count.) The most useful reasoning strategy in the workup of a patient with an increased WBC count involves (1) a diagnostic workup toward the most *probable* diagnostic possibility or (2) a workup toward the most *important* diagnostic possibility (*"diagnosis you can't afford to miss"*). In practical terms, this poses the question of making a distinction between increased WBC due to *reactive leukocytosis* (very common) or due to a primary *hematologic disorder* (relatively rare, but serious).

Since there are numerous reasons for an increase in WBC (physical and/or emotional stimuli, infections, inflammations, drugs, toxins, etc.), the approach to identification of these disorders is best accomplished by a carefully taken history and physical exam. Particular attention should be given to the disclosure of lymphadenopathy and splenomegaly. The most important hematologic entities to consider are *acute leukemia(s), chronic leukemia(s)* and *myeloproliferative syndrome*. Examination of the peripheral blood and bone marrow aspirate/biopsy are the two most important diagnostic procedures in differentiating between reactive leukocytosis and primary hematologic disorder. If examination of the peripheral blood does not disclose immature cells, the next step should be to determine which blood cells are responsible for the high WBC (i.e., whether one is dealing with neutrophilia, lymphocytosis, eosino-

philia, basophilia, or monocytosis). In the vast majority of cases, secondary reasons will be responsible for this abnormality. Sometimes one may see WBC in a range of 50,000–100,000/mm³ (50–100 × 10⁹/L) (usually neutrophilia). This type of leukemoid reaction, commonly seen in severe infections, inflammation, and tumors, should be differentiated from *chronic myeloid leukemia* (CML). The most useful test in this case is *leukocyte alkaline phosphatase* (LAP), which is typically low or absent in CML, and normal or high in other conditions. Alternatively, one may look for a *Ph chromosome* or *bcr/abl gene-rearrangement*, which are positive in 95% and 97% of CML cases, respectively. It should also be mentioned that finding Döhle bodies or cytoplasmatic

Table 21-1. The 95% Confidence Limits for the Leukocyte and Leukocyte Differential Counts[a]

Total leukocytes	3,931–10,060
Total neutrophils	1,874–6,847
Lymphocytes	1,162–3,516
Eosinophils	12.5–591
Monocytes	191–859
Basophils	0–143

[a] Data from three studies, as presented in Shapiro and Greenfield. Data expressed in count/μl. Note that decision levels in algorithms are greater than 95% confidence values.

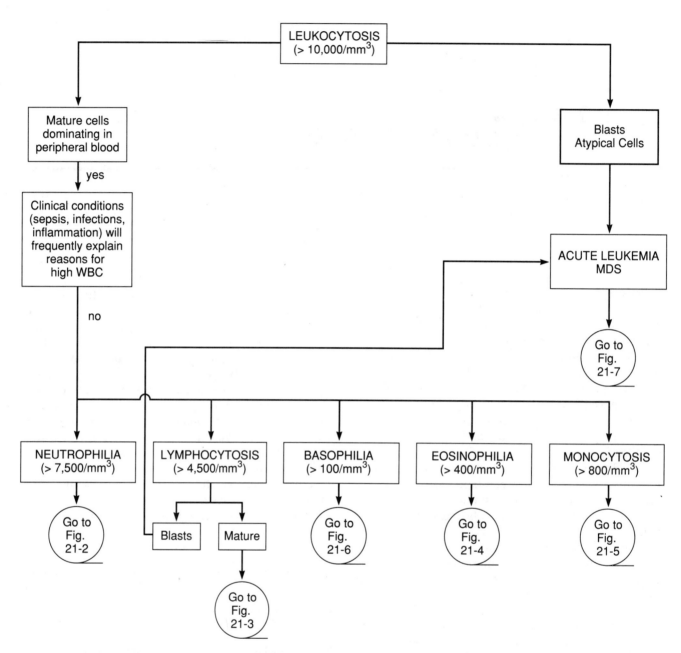

Fig. 21-1. Diagnostic approach to leukocytosis. The major clinical problem is the distinction between *reactive* leukocytosis (the most probable cause) and *primary* hematologic disease (the most serious disorder, "diagnosis you can't afford to miss"). A careful history and physical exam are of crucial importance in identifying the causes of reactive leukocytosis.

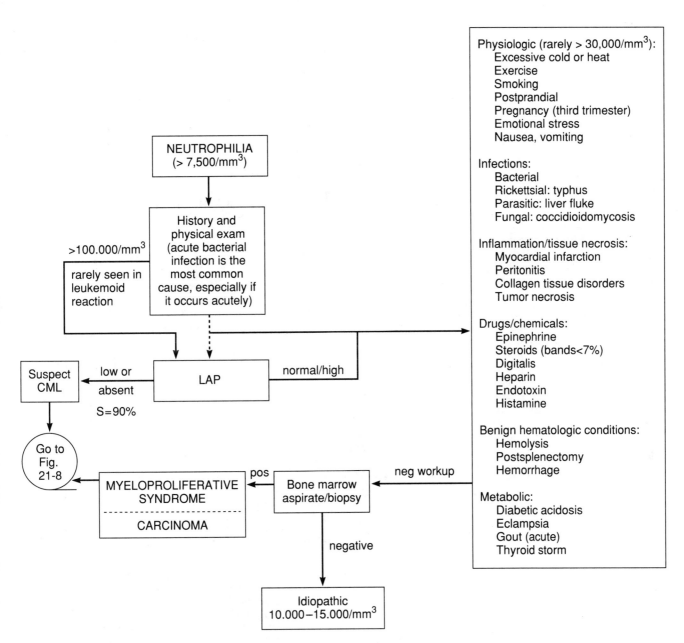

Fig. 21-2. Diagnostic approach to neutrophilia. The major clinical problem is the distinction between *reactive* leukocytosis (the most probable cause) and *primary* hematologic disease (the most serious disorder, "diagnosis you can't afford to miss"). LAP is 90% sensitive in a diagnosis of CML—the most important differential diagnostic consideration.

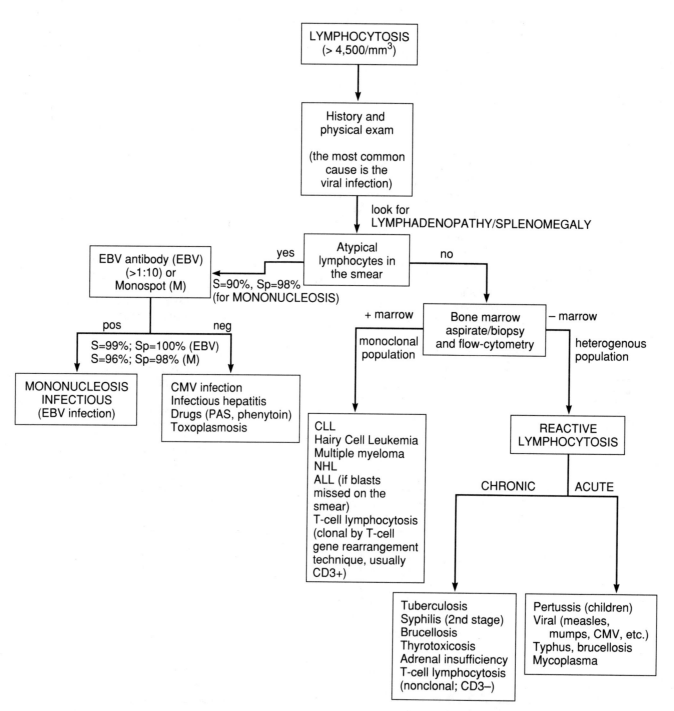

Fig. 21-3. Diagnostic approach to lymphocytosis. The major clinical problem is the distinction between *reactive* leukocytosis (the most probable cause) and *primary* hematologic disease (the most serious disorder, "diagnosis you can't afford to miss"). Flowcytometry is an expensive test, but offers the proof of monoclonality—virtually pathognomonic for malignancy—which, in the end, makes it a cost-effective test.

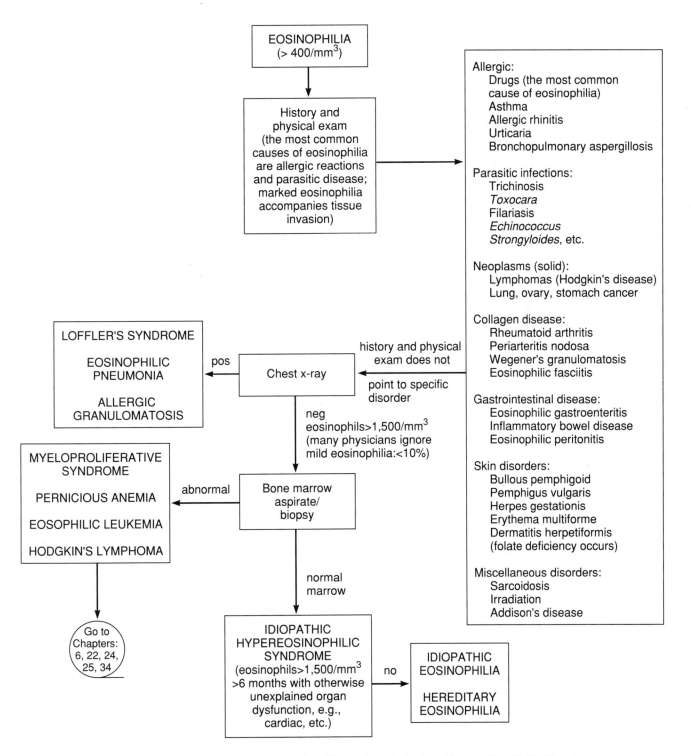

Fig. 21-4. Diagnostic approach to eosinophilia. The major clinical problem is the distinction between *reactive* leukocytosis (the most probable cause) and *primary* hematologic disease (the most serious disorder, "diagnosis you can't afford to miss"). Always rule out drugs as the cause of eosinophilia before diagnostic workup is started.

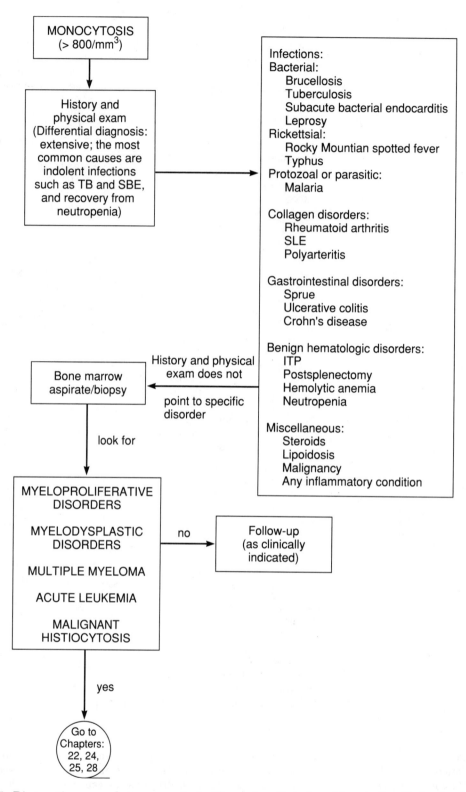

Fig. 21-5. Diagnostic approach to monocytosis. The major clinical problem is the distinction between *reactive* leukocytosis (the most probable cause) and *primary* hematologic disease (the most serious disorder, "diagnosis you can't afford to miss").

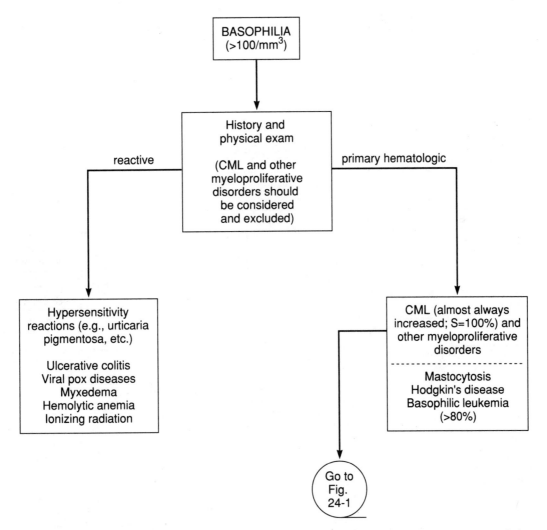

Fig. 21-6. Diagnostic approach to basophilia. The major clinical problem is the distinction between *reactive* leukocytosis (the most probable cause) and *primary* hematologic disease (the most serious disorder, "diagnosis you can't afford to miss"). Think of CML first when you encounter basophilia (S‑100%).

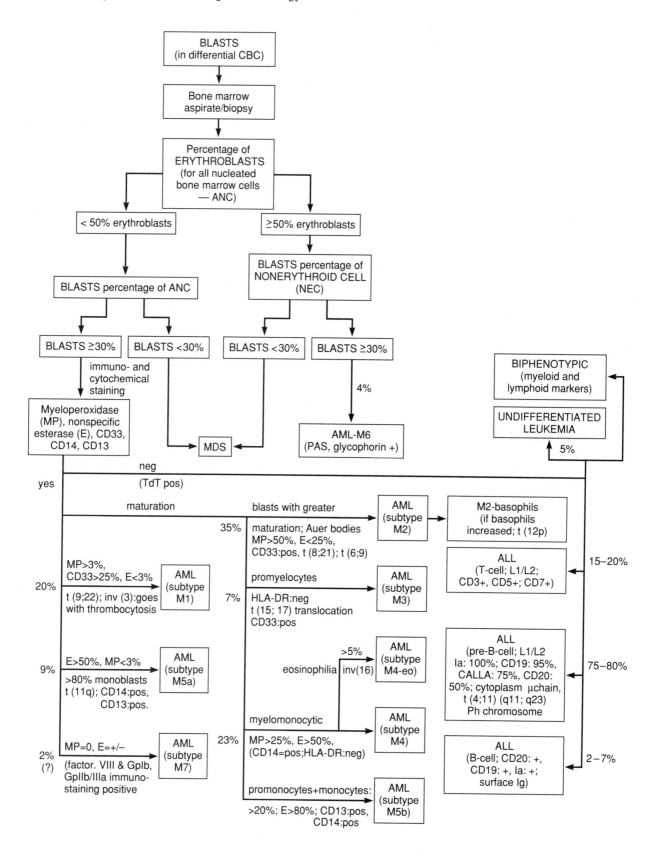

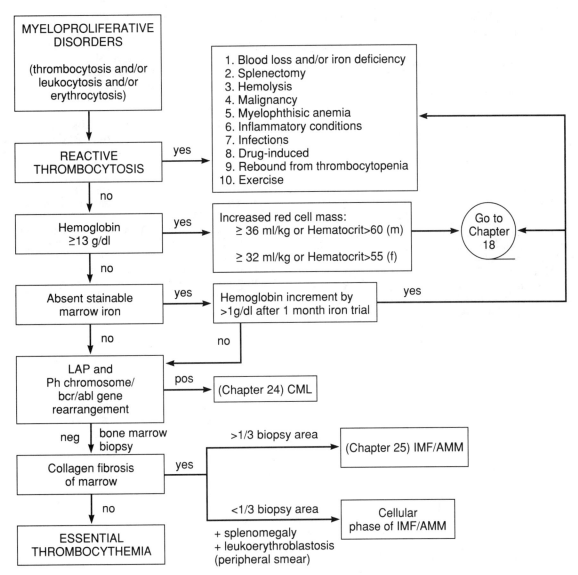

Fig. 21-8. Polycythemia Vera Study Group algorithm for diagnosis of myeloproliferative disorders (From Williams JD et al.: Hematology, 4th Ed. McGraw-Hill, New York, 1990, with permission). (See individual chapters for further discussions of these problems.)

Fig. 21-7. Algorithm for diagnosis of acute leukemia. The most important clinical issue is the distinction between MDS, AML, and ALL. The French-American-British Cooperative Group has developed an algorithm based upon morphologic and cytochemical features for the diagnosis of AL. Morphology alone can help us correctly make this distinction in about 70% of cases; with additional cytochemistry, the diagnostic rate is increased to 86%; and with the use of immunological markers, the accuracy rate has increased to greater than 95%. Note that the most specific morphological marker for AML is the finding of Auer rods, with a specificity of almost 100%, but a very low sensitivity (20%). Immunological staining is of key importance for the subclassification of ALL. In about 60% of cases cytogenetic abnormalities may be identified; their diagnostic value is still limited, although in certain cases they may provide us with some information (e.g., t(15;17) in diagnosing of M3). This figure illustrates the most characteristic karyotype abnormalities to show the concept of emerging *morphologic-immunologic-cytogenetic* classification of acute leukemias.

vacuoles in neutrophils is almost pathognomonic for infections. Figures 21-1–21-6 show a logical strategy for the workup of high WBC. The French-American-British (FAB) Cooperative Group has defined a strategy for cases when acute leukemia or myelodysplastic disorder is suspected (Fig. 21-7). A Polycythemia Vera Study Group has created a set of production rules for the workup of myeloproliferative disorders (Fig. 21-8).

Suggested Readings

Bennett JM, Catovsky D, Daniel T, et al.: The morphological classification of acute lymphoblastic leukemia:concordance among observers and clinical correlations. Br J Haematol 47:553, 1981

Bennett JM, Catovsky D, Daniel MT, et al.: Criteria for the diagnosis of acute leukemia of megakaryocyte lineage (M7). A report of the French-American-British Cooperative Group. Ann Intern Med 103:460, 1985

Bennett JM, Catovsky D, Daniel MT, et al.: Proposed revised criteria for the classification of acute myeloid leukemia. A report of the French-American-British Cooperative Group. Ann Intern Med 103:626, 1985

First MIC Cooperative Study Group. Morphologic, immunologic, and cytogenetic (MIC) working classification of the acute lymphoblastic leukemias. Cancer Genet Cytogenet 23:189, 1986

Iland HJ, Laszlo J: Myeloproliferative disorders: Polycythemia Vera, Essential Thrombocythemia and Idiopathic/Agnogenic Myeloid Metaplasia. In Hoogstraten B (ed.): Hematologic Malignancies. Springer-Verlag, Berlin, 1986

Krause JR, Penchansky L, Contis L, Kaplan SS: Flow cytometry in the diagnosis of acute leukemia. Am J Clin Pathol 89:341, 1988

Meeting Report. Morphologic, immunologic, and cytogenetic (MIC) working classification of the acute myeloid leukaemias. Br J Haematol 68:487, 1988

Shapiro MF, Greenfield S: The complete blood count and leukocyte differential count. An approach to their rational application. Ann Intern Med 106:65, 1987

22 | Acute Myeloid Leukemia

Acute myeloid leukemia (AML) is a clonal disorder of hematopoietic cells that, until 20 years ago, was uniformly fatal. AML accounts for 80% of all acute leukemia in adults and increases in frequency with age, with an average incidence of 3–5 per 100,000 population, but as high as 15 per 100,000 in the eighth and ninth decades. In the majority of patients it arises de novo, but in a small subset AML is preceded by de novo or chemotherapy-induced myelodysplasia, and is referred to as *secondary AML*.

The diagnosis of AML is usually made after either *quantitative* (high or low white blood cells (WBC), see Chapters 21 and 27) or *qualitative* (immature cells, see Chapter 21, Fig. 21-7) changes in a complete blood count (CBC) are found. Clinical manifestations of AML are related to anemia, neutropenia, and thrombocytopenia due to suppression of normal hematopoiesis. Anemia, thrombocytopenia, and blasts are almost always detected at diagnosis. However, bone marrow biopsy/aspiration is the key diagnostic procedure for the diagnosis of AML, and should be performed if AML is suspected (gold standard test). Formal criteria for diagnosis are defined in terms of *production rules* by the French-American-British (FAB) Cooperative Group (see Chapter 21, Fig. 21-7).

The most important elements involved in the *reasoning strategy* regarding the management of AML are (1) prediction of the *course* of the disease, and (2) prediction of the *response* to treatment. The reasoning strategy, in fact, is *probabilistic*. If left untreated, the median survival of patients with AML is about 6 weeks, with only 3% of patients surviving 1 year. This high probability of demise in AML patients lead to the formulation of the clinical rule that *all* patients with AML should be treated. Treatment should be initiated within 24–48 hours of diagnosis ("AML is a hematologic emergency").

Probability of the response to therapy will dictate the choice of treatment, which will, in turn, depend on the exact *morphologic diagnosis* (M3 *vs* all other subtypes) and the *risk factors* present (Fig. 22-1 and box below). Treatment of AML involves *induction chemotherapy* (eradication of leukemic cells below clinically detectable level) with ara-C (cytosine ar-

---

Prognostic Factors in Acute Myeloid Leukemia

Very Important
M3 subtype (favorable)
Age (>60: unfavorable)
Chromosome abnormalities:
    (8;21)—high CR and long survival
    16q22, t(15;17)—average CR and survival
    t(9;11)—short CR and survival
    12p−,5q−,+13 sole, +8 sole, inv 3—low induction rate
Secondary AML (unfavorable)

Less Important[a]
Other FAB subtypes (M4–M7, unfavorable)
Performance status (>50%, favorable)
WBC count (>50 × 10^9/L, unfavorable)
Labelling index (high, favorable)
Presence of Auer rods (favorable)

---

[a] Many other factors were identified; however, they have not been consistently reproduced in all studies.

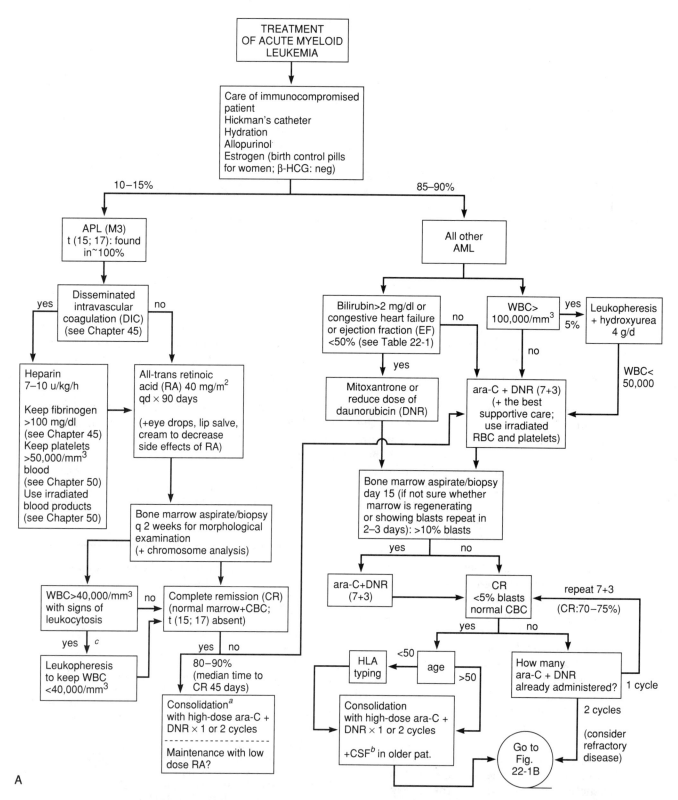

A

Fig. 22-1 (A and B). Treatment of AML. *Probabilistic reasoning strategy* coupled with *risk/benefit estimate* dominates management of adult AML. The initial choice of treatment will depend on morphologic subtype (M3 *vs* others in FAB classification). The choice of post-remission therapy is more controversial and dictated by the probability of response and the estimate of mortality/morbidity associated with each available management strategy.

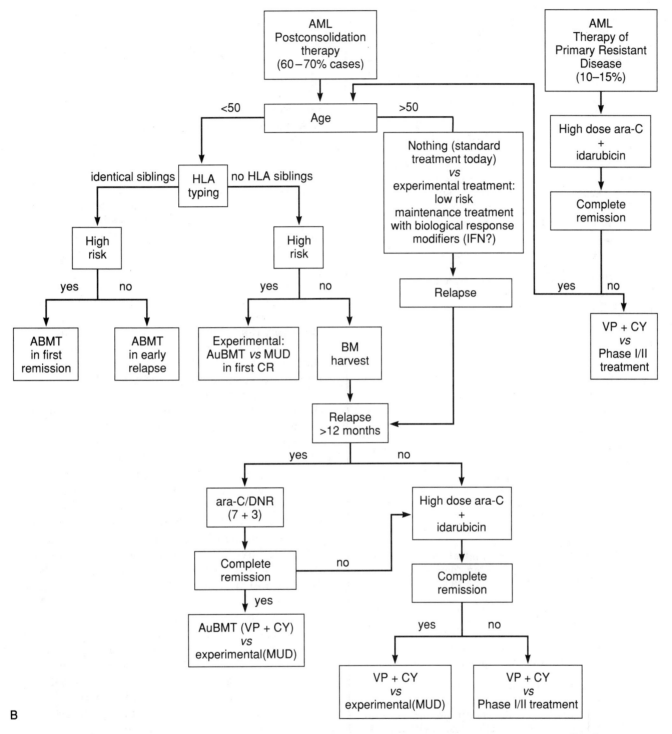

Fig. 22-1 *(Continued)*. AML is a hematologic *emergency,* and timely use of supportive care (antibiotics, blood products, corrections of hydromineral disbalance) is as important as the choice of a proper chemotherapeutic regimen. (Abbreviations (see box in Chapter 22): MUD, matched unrelated donor; CSF, colony stimulating factors (e.g., G-CSF and GM-CSF; AuBMT, autologous bone marrow transplantation; ABMT, allogeneic bone marrow transplantation.) [a] Authors' bias (extrapolated from available data); [b] Preliminary data (ara-C reduction for age: 1.5 g/m²); [c] Recommended by some authors; others would use hydroxyurea or continue same initial therapy.

Drug Doses and Other Treatment Measures in Management of AML

Cytosine arabinoside + daunomycin (ara-C + DNR, 7 + 3):
  Ara-C 100 mg/m^2 continuous IV × 7 days
  DNR 45 mg/m^2 IV on days 1, 2, 3
    or
  Mitoxantrone 12 mg/m^2 IV × 3 days
    or
  Ara-C + idarubicin 13 mg/m^2/d × 3 (most recent study suggests that this combination is superior to ara-C + DNR regimen)

All-trans Retinoic Acid:
  40 mg/m^2 PO daily × 90 days

High-dose ara-C (HiD-ara-C) + DNR:
  Ara-C 1.5–3.0 g/m^2 IV q 12 hours × 12 (infusion over 1 hour) (1.5 g/m^2 if > 50 in age)
  DNR 30 mg/m^2 IV on days 7, 8, 9
  Decadron eye drops qid × 10 days

High-dose ara-C + idarubicin:
  Ara-C 1 g/m^2 IV q 12 hours × 6 doses
  Idarubicin 8–12 mg/m^2 IV × 3 days
  Decadron eye drops qid × 5 days

Etoposide + Cyclophosphamide (VP + CY):
  Etoposide 4.0 g/m^2 continuous IV × 72 hours (not to exceed 2 mg/minute)
  Cyclophosphamide 50 mg/kg IV on days 4, 5, 6, 7
  Vigorous hydration with Cy to keep urine flow > 100 ml/hr until 24 hrs after chemotherapy

Supportive measures:
  Allopurinol—300 mg/day PO till aplasia (tumor lysis syndrome prevention)
  Anti-emetics before chemotherapy (e.g., decadron 10 mg IV × 3 days)
  Ativan 1 mg IV q 6 hours prn (no IM injection in thrombocytopenia!)
  Estrogen or birth control pills in women to prevent menstrual bleeding (danger of exsanguination): norethindrone 10 mg qd till platelets > 50 × 10^9/L
  Keep platelets > 20 × 10^9/L (go to Chapter 50) (use irradiated leukopoor platelets, preferably from single donor)
  Keep hemoglobin > 10 g/dl (use leukopoor and CMV negative RBC products) (see Chapter 51)
  Antibiotics at the first sign of infection (or temperature ≥ 38°C) (go to Chapter 30)
  Lab monitoring CBC, creatinine, and electrolytes daily; liver function tests twice a week

---

abinoside) and DNR (daunomycin) (7 + 3), which is as effective as more dose-intensive therapies but less toxic (complete remission (CR) = 70–80%). This treatment should be used in all subtypes of AML except the M3 subtype (acute promyelocytic leuke-mia). The use of All-trans retinoic acid in *acute promyelocytic leukemia* (APL) results in 80–90% CR rates without marrow aplasia, and has revolutionized therapy of this subset of AML. Reestablishment of normal bone marrow morphology with <5% blasts and normal peripheral blood counts is defined as CR, and occurs in 70–80% of patients.

A major decision dilemma exists regarding *postremission therapy* (Fig. 22-1B) aims to eradicate clinically undetectable leukemic cells. With CR rates of 70–80% from induction therapy in standard risk patients, the remaining task is to improve cure rates by preventing early relapse. The options for post remission therapy include* (1) *consolidation/intensification*, (2) *allogeneic bone marrow transplantation* (ABMT), and (3) *autologous bone marrow transplantation* (AuBMT).

A recent trial indicated that ABMT, in first remission, did not offer a survival advantage over intensive post-remission consolidation chemotherapy. However, relapse rates and treatment-related mortalities were substantially different, which indicates that determination of the *risk/benefit* ratio in each individual case should guide treatment choice. In terms of mortality and overall disease-free survival (DFS), *consolidation* therapy carries a mortality risk of about 5–10%. A projected 5 year DFS of 40–50% for high dose ara-C + DNR, and 15–20% for standard chemotherapy (7 + 3) have been reported respectively. Overall, death risk for ABMT is between 15–35%, with a projected 5 year DFS exceeding 40–50% for young patients. Relapse rate after ABMT is the lowest of all other therapeutic modalities. However, most patients with AML are >50 yrs, and only 35% will have HLA-identical siblings. Thus, only 10–15% of AML patients will be eligible for ABMT. The optimal timing of ABMT in standard-risk patients is probably early in the first relapse. AuBMT carries a death risk similar to chemotherapy. Three years DFS is only 20–25% at this time, due to high relapse rates, but is slightly better than standard chemotherapy alone. However, because the 3 year DFS of AuBMT in first CR is similar to that achieved with intensification, an optimal timing for AuBMT may be during second remission. Fig. 22-1B shows an interpretation of available data.

The prognosis of AML with modern therapy has resulted in improved survival—a median of 12 months and 25–30% long-term survival in those pa-

---

* It is clear that some form of postremission therapy is needed. If no treatment is administered, long-term survival is virtually zero. If standard maintenance (but low toxic treatment) is given, long-term survival is about 10–15% only.

Table 22-1. Dose Modification with Hepatic Dysfunction

Drug	Bilirubin < 1.5 mg/dl and SGOT < 60 IU (%)	Bilirubin = 1.5–3.0 and SGOT = 60–180 (%)	Bilirubin = 3–5 and SGOT > 180 (%)	Bilirubin > 5
Cyclophosphamide	100	100	75	Omit
Methotrexate	100	100	75	Omit
Daunorubicin	100	75	50	Omit
Doxorubicin	100	50	25	Omit
Vinblastine	100	50	Omit	Omit
Vincristine	100	50	Omit	Omit
Etoposide	100	50	Omit	Omit

tients achieving CR. The major causes of death are infection (immunocompromised patient) and bleeding (15%), underscoring the importance of *supportive* therapy in AML patients (see Chapters 30, 50, and 51).

Suggested Readings

Appelbaum FR, Fisher LD, Thomas ED: Chemotherapy *vs* marrow transplantation for adults with acute nonlymphocytic leukemia: a five-year follow-up. Blood 72:179, 1988

Butturini A and Gale RP: Annotation: chemotherapy *vs* transplantation in acute leukemia. Br J Haematol 73:1, 1989

Champlin R and Gale RP: Bone marrow transplantation for acute leukemia: recent advances and comparison with alternative strategies. Semin Hematol 24:55, 1987

Chen ZX, Xue YQ, Zhang R, Tao RF, et al.: A clinical and experimental study on all-trans retinoic acid-treated acute promyelocytic leukemia patients. Blood 78:1413, 1991

Mayer RJ: Current chemotherapeutic treatment approaches to the management of previously untreated adults with de novo acute myelogenous leukemia. Semin Oncol 14:384, 1987

Reiffers J, Gaspard MH, Maraninchi D, et al.: Comparison of allogeneic or autologous bone marrow transplantation and chemotherapy in patients with acute myeloid leukemia in first remission: a prospective controlled trial. Br J Haematol 72:57, 1989

Schiffer CA and Lee EJ: Approaches to the therapy of relapsed acute myeloid leukemia. Oncology 3:23, 1989

Schiller GJ, Nimer SD, Territo MC, et al.: BMT *vs* high-dose cytarabine-based consolidation chemotherapy for acute myelogenous leukemia in first remission. J Clin Oncol 10:41, 1992

23 | Adult Acute Lymphoblastic Leukemia*

Acute lymphoblastic leukemia (ALL) is a malignant disorder of hematopoietic cells with an overall incidence similar to AML (3–5 per 100,000 population), but with a shift to younger patients, being the most common malignancy under the age of 15. ALL accounts for approximately 15–25% of all adult leukemia.

The diagnosis of ALL is usually made after either *quantitative* (high or low white blood cells (WBC), see Chapters 21, 27) or *qualitative* (immature cells, see Chapter 21, Fig. 21-7) changes in the CBC are found. Clinical manifestations of AML are related to anemia, neutropenia, and thrombocytopenia due to suppression of normal hematopoiesis. Anemia, thrombocytopenia, and blasts are almost always detected at diagnosis. In about 30% of adult patients, the initial WBC is less $< 5 \times 10^9$/L, making detection of blasts more difficult. Bone marrow biopsy/aspiration is the key diagnostic procedure for diagnosis of ALL, and should be performed if this diagnosis is suspected (gold standard test). Formal criteria for diagnosis are defined in terms of *production rules* by the French-American-British (FAB) Cooperative Group (see Chapter 21, Fig. 21-7). Those (morphologic and cytochemical) criteria must be combined with further immunological and cytogenetic information. After immunologic subtyping,

about 90% of ALL should be classifiable: common ALL approximately 50–60%; T-ALL approximately 20–25%; B-ALL approximately 5%; mixed-ALL approximately 1%, and the rest unclassifiable (null-ALL).

The most important elements involved in *reasoning strategy* regarding the management of ALL are (1) prediction of the course of disease, and (2) prediction of the response to treatment. Reasoning strategy, in fact, is *probabilistic*. The high probability of the demise of patients with ALL leads to the formulation of a clinical rule: all patients with ALL should be treated, and treatment should be initiated within 24–48 hours after diagnosis ("ALL is a hematologic emergency").

Treatment strategy consists of *induction* (eradication of leukemia detectable by conventional techniques), *consolidation/intensification* (elimination of clinically undetectable leukemia), *maintenance* (pre-

---

* This chapter is influenced by Professor D. Hoelzer's lecture at the 33rd annual meeting of the American Society for Hematology. Professor Hoelzer also kindly provided us with the latest protocols for treatment of adult ALL (see boxes on pp. 108 and 111). Although the final results of these protocols are yet to be published, we have incorporated them here because of the initial, promising results and the overall disappointment with old protocols.

> **The Most Important (Adverse) Prognostic Factors for Predicting Course of Disease and Selection of Treatment Strategy in Acute Lymphoblastic Leukemia**
>
> ---
>
> Age > 35
> WBC $> 30 \times 10^9$/L
> Time to remission > 4 weeks
> Chromosome abnormalities [t(9;22) and t(4;11)]
> B-ALL
> Hybrid ALL
> Pre-T (?)

Chemotherapy Regimen for Treatment of Acute Lymphoblastic Leukemia (ALL)

Regimen for the treatment of adult T and standard-risk ALL

Induction (weeks 1–8):[a]
Phase I:
- Prednisone 60 mg/m² PO days 1–29
- Asparaginase 5,000 U/m² IV days 15–29
- Vincristine 2 mg IV days 1, 8, 15, 22
- Daunorubicin 45 mg/m² IV days 1, 8, 15, 22

Phase II:
- Cyclophosphamide 650 mg/m² IV days 29, 43, 57
- Cytosine arabinoside 75 mg/m² IV days 31–34, 38–41, 45–48, 52–55
- Mercaptopurine 60 mg/m² PO days 29–57

CNS prophylaxis (when patient is in remission):
- Cranial irradiation (24 Gy over 4 weeks; 30 Gy in primary involvement of CNS)
- Methotrexate 15 mg IT once a week during Phase II of induction therapy (i.e., days 31, 38, 45, 52 or after complete remission is achieved)

Consolidation therapy (weeks 13, 17 or 31, 35 after induction therapy)[a]
- Cytosine arabinoside 75 mg/m² IV days 1–5
- VM26 60 mg/m² IV (vindesine) days 1–5

Maintenance therapy (weeks 39–142)[b]
- Mercaptopurin 60 mg/m² PO daily
- Methotrexate 20 mg/m² IV (PO) once a week

[a] If remission is not achieved, reinduce with the same regimen at weeks 21–26.
[b] Dose adjustment for mercaptopurin and methotrexate (aim is to keep WBC <3.5 and >2.5 and platelets >75):

Platelets (×10⁹/L)	>2.5 (%)	2.0–2.5 (%)	1.5–2.0 (%)	<1.5 (%)
>100	100	75	33	0
75–100	75	75	33	0
50–75	33	33	33	0
<50	0	0	0	0

WBC (×10⁹/L) spans the four percentage columns above.

Chemotherapy Regimen for Treatment of Acute Lymphocytic Leukemia (ALL)

Regimen for the treatment of adult high-risk ALL (pH +, null, or mixed ALL)

Induction (weeks 1–8):
Phase I:
- Prednisone 60 mg/m² PO days 1–29
- Asparaginase 5,000 U/m² IV days 15–29
- Vincristine 2 mg IV days 1, 8, 15, 22
- Daunorubicin 45 mg/m² IV days 1, 9, 15, 22

Phase II:
- Cyclophosphamide 650 mg/m² IV days 29, 43, 57
- Cytosine arabinoside 75 mg/m² IV days 31–34, 38–41, 45–48, 52–55
- Mercaptopurine 60 mg/m² PO days 29–57

CNS prophylaxis (when patient is in remission):
- Cranial irradiation (24 Gy over 4 weeks; 30 Gy in primary involvement of CNS)
- Methotrexate 15 mg IT once a week during Phase II of induction therapy (i.e., days 31, 38, 45, 52 or after complete remission is achieved)

Consolidation therapy[a]
Arm A (week 13):
- High-dose cytosine arabinoside 1 g/m² IV days bid in 3-hour infusions days 1–4
- Mitoxantrone 10 mg/m² IV days 2–5
Arm B (weeks 13, 15, 17; see Table 23-1 for high-dose methotrexate administration)
- High-dose methotexate 1,500 mg/m² IV day 1
- Asparaginase 10,000 U/m² IV day 2

Maintenance therapy (weeks 39–142; see box above for dose adjustment)
- Mercaptopurin 60 mg/m² PO daily
- Methotrexate 20 mg/m² IV (PO) once a week

[a] Ongoing study

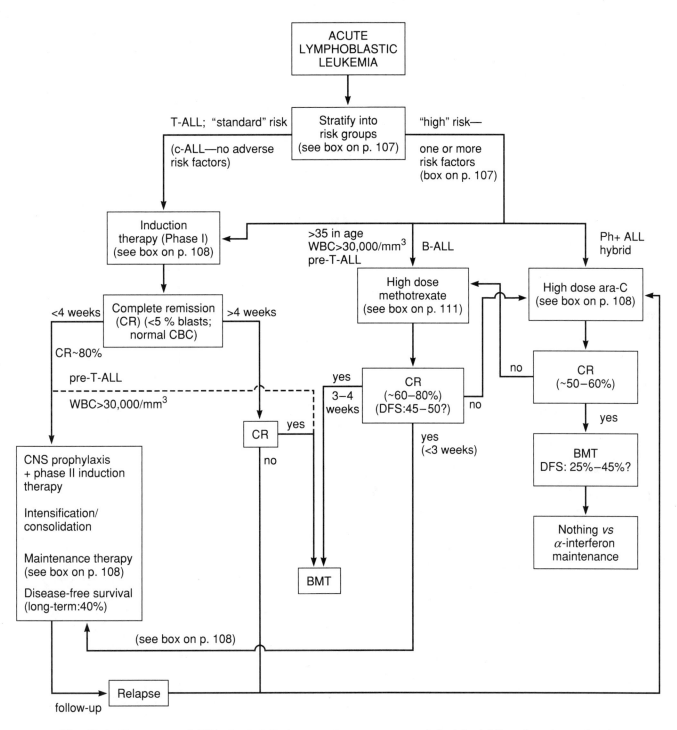

Fig. 23-1. Treatment of ALL. *Probabilistic reasoning strategy* coupled with *risk/benefit estimate* dominates management of adult ALL. The initial choice of therapy will depend on assigning the patient to a specific "risk group"; this reflects our estimate of the course of disease and its response to therapy, which is individualized according to these estimates. ALL is a hematologic *emergency*, and timely use of supportive care (antibiotics, blood products, corrections of hydromineral imbalance) is equally as important as the choice of a proper chemotherapeutic regimen (see also chapter on the treatment of AML).

Table 23-1. High-dose Methotrexate with Leukovorin Rescue

Methotrexate (MTX) Administration	Day	Time	Time Point After MTX Start	MTX Serum Concentration Determination	Leukovorin Doses Depending on Serum MTX Levels
200 mg/m² IV (30 min)	1	14.00	0		
1,300 mg/m² IV (23 ½ hrs.)					
End of continuous IV infusion (give with 3 liters of fluid 5% glucose with 40 mEq of NaHCO₃ + 20 mEq KCl). Forced diuresis with furosemide 40 mg after 6 and 12 hours to titrate pH > 7.2)	2	14.00	24		
	3	2.00	36		
		8.00 "	42	× if Serum MTX <0.5 μM	Rescue 30 mg/m² IV if Serum MTX >0.5–5 μM
		14.00	48	30 mg/m² PO	50 mg/m² IV
		20.00	54	15 mg/m² PO	50 mg/m² IV
	4	2.00	60	5 mg/m² PO	50 mg/m² IV } every 6 hours × 4
					50 mg/m² IV
		10.00 "	68	× if Serum MTX <0.1 μM	if Serum MTX >0.1 μM
		16.00	74	5 mg/m² PO	30 mg/m² IV
		20.00	78	5 mg/m² PO	30 mg/m² IV } every 6 hours × 4
		22.00	80		
	5	4.00	86		30 mg/m² IV
					30 mg/m² IV

Chemotherapy Regimen for Treatment of Acute Lymphoblastic Leukemia (ALL)

Regimen for the treatment of adult B-ALL)

Prephase:
  Cyclophosphamide 200 mg/m^2 IV days 1–5
  Prednisone 60 mg/m^2 PO days 1–5

Block A:
  Vincristine 2 mg IV day 1
  High-dose methotrexate 1,500 mg/m^2 in 24 hour infusion day 1[a]
  Ifosphamid 800 mg/m^2 1 hour infusion days 1–5
  VM26 100 mg/m^2 1 hour infusion days 4–5
  Cytosine arabinoside 150 mg/m^2 q 12 hours as 1-hour infusion days 4, 5

  Dexamethasone 10 mg/m^2 PO days 1–5

  Methotrexate 15 mg ⎫
  Ara-C 40 mg   ⎬ IT days 1–5
  Dexamethasone 4 mg ⎭

Block B (after 16 days of rest; start schedule on Monday):
  Vincristine 2 mg IV day 1
  High-dose methotrexate 1,500 mg/m^2 in 24-hour infusion days 1[a]
  Cyclophosphamide 200 mg/m^2 IV days 1–5
  Adriamycin 25 mg/m^2 IV (15 minutes) days 4, 5

  Dexamethasone 10mg/m^2 PO days 1–5

  Methotrexate 15 mg ⎫
  Ara-C 40 mg   ⎬ IT days 1–5
  Dexamethasone 4 mg ⎭

CNS Prophylaxis:
  Skull irradiation with 24 Gy after Block B therapy

Treatment of CNS Involvement:
  Skull irradiation and irradiation of the remaining neuroaxis plus therapy with methotrexate, cytosine arabinoside, and dexamethasone until liquor clears

---

[a] See Table 23-1.

vention of clinical relapse), and *central nervous system (CNS) prophylaxis* (reduction of the risk of CNS relapse). Although this treatment strategy is physiologically sound, it has still not been empirically verified in controlled trials; uncontrolled experience, however, favors this approach.

The choice of specific therapy is dictated by the probability of response to it, which, in turn, depends on prognostic factors (see box on p. 107) associated with a particular ALL. The major decision dilemma relates to the role of bone marrow transplant in first remission. Recent analysis of data shows that BMT offers no advantage over chemotherapy, but that there is a certain subset of high-risk adult patients who may benefit from BMT in first remission. Deciding which treatment strategy to choose then depends on the classification of ALL according to "high risk" vs "standard risk" (Fig. 23-1 and box on p. 108). Probabilistic estimates again dominate clinical decision making in the management of adult patients with ALL.

The treatment of ALL with modern therapy has resulted in an improved prognosis for survival, with >70–80% of patients achieving remission and about 35–45% of patients showing long-term survival. As in AML, the major causes of death are infection (immunocompromised patient) and bleeding, underscoring the importance of *supportive* therapy in ALL patients (see Chapters 30, 50).

Suggested Readings

Butturini A, Gale RP: Chemotherapy versus transplantation in acute leukaemia. Br J Haematol 72:1, 1989

Champlin R, Gale RP: Acute lymphoblastic leukemia: recent advances in biology and therapy. Blood 73:2051, 1989

Herzig RH, Bortin MM, Barrett A, et al.: Bone marrow transplantation in high-risk acute lymphoblastic leukemia in first and second remission. Lancet I:786, 1987

Hoelzer D, Gale RP: Acute lymphoblastic leukemia in adults: recent progress, future directions. Semin Hematol 24:27, 1987

Hoelzer D, Theil E, Loffler H, et al.: Prognostic factors in a multicenter study for treatment of acute lymphoblastic leukemia in adults. Blood 71:123, 1988

Horowitz MM, Messerer D, Hoelzer D, et al.: Chemotherapy compared with bone marrow transplantation for adults with acute lymphoblastic leukemia in first remission. Ann Intern Med 115:13, 1991

24 Chronic Myelogenous Leukemia

Chronic myelogenous leukemia (CML) accounts for about 20% of all leukemia cases, with a death rate of about 1.5 per 100,000 population. The disease is rather rare among the young, with only 10% of cases occurring between the ages of 5 and 20. The median age of diagnosis is about 43 years. Typical clinical features include splenomegaly (S = 90%), neutrophilia, basophilia, and thrombocytosis with hypercellular bone marrow. Specific laboratory findings include a low score of leukocyte alkaline phosphatase (LAP) (found low only in PNH, and sometimes in myelodysplastic syndrome (MDS), idiopathic thrombocytopenia purpura (ITP), infectious mononucleosis, pernicious anemia and congenital hypophosphatasia), Philadelphia chromosome (Ph), found in 90–95% of cases of CML, and bcr-abl gene rearrangement. Only a minority of patients (3–5%) are *both* Ph chromosome negative *and* do not show breakpoint cluster region rearrangement (bcr).

The natural *history* of CML is characterized by an evolution of the disease from a chronic phase through an accelerated to a terminal phase of acute leukemia, the so-called blast crisis or blast transformation. Patients with CML may live anywhere from a few months to 14 years, with a median survival rate of between 2–4 years.

Traditional *treatment* of CML has been with chemotherapy agents such as busulfan or hydroxyurea. This treatment, however, does not lead to cytogenetic remission (Ph chromosome does not disappear), and thus does not change the natural history of the disease. Currently, bone marrow transplantation (BMT) is considered the only possible curative treatment for CML. This is not a risk-free procedure, however, since it has a mortality rate of between 20–30% (and up to 46% in some series). *Optimal timing* of BMT becomes, therefore, the key element in the management of patients with CML. Figure 24-1 shows a method for determination of this time-threshold for BMT in *individual patients* (for a *group* of CML patients, taken as a *whole*, some data indicate that optimal timing would be within the first year of diagnosis). Recently, there have been reports of successful remission induction (hematologic + cytogenetic) with α-interferon. Initial studies suggest that this can convert to survival advantage (median survival of 62 months *vs* 39 months for conservative therapy in MD Anderson series). Figure 24-2 outlines details of clinical management of CML.

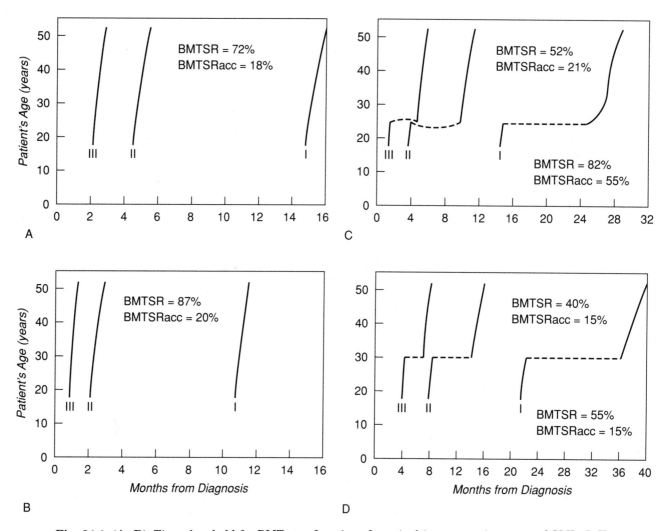

Fig. 24-1. (A–D) Time-threshold for BMT as a function of survival in prognostic groups of CML (I, II, III), BMT success rates in chronic cases (BMTSR), and accelerated/blastic (BMTSRacc) phases of disease and patient's age. To determine optimal timing of BMT in an *individual patient,* first enquire about results for BMT of the particular center you are referring your patient to (some results reported in the literature are shown elsewhere in this figure). Second, determine the prognostic group of CML for your patient. Third, draw a line from your patient's age on ordinate to the corresponding prognostic group, and then from this intersection draw a vertical line to the abscissa. Read this value as the optimal timing of BMT after CML is diagnosed. Prognostic groups are determined according to Sokal et al.: Blood 63:789, 1984: A = $\exp^{.116}$ × (age–43.4); B = .345 × (spleen size(cm)–7.51); C = .188 × (platelet/700)^2–.563; D = 8.86 × 10^{-2} × (% blast–2.1). G = A + B + C + D. If G < .78, then patient is in group I; if G ≥ .78 ≤ 1.3, then patient is in group II; if G > 1.3, then patient is in group III. (From Denic S, Djulbegovic B, Ridzanovic Z: Period Biol 91:391, 1989, with permission.)

Fig. 24-2. Treatment of chronic myelogenous leukemia (CML). Estimates of the *risk/benefit* of different treatment options dominates decision making in the treatment of CML. The major decision is whether to perform the only known curative procedure—bone marrow transplantation (BMT)—or not. A new element appears in the management of CML: determination of the optimal timing of this curative but high-risk procedure (see Fig. 24-1). Note that the age cutoff of when to offer a standard treatment *vs* BMT or interferon therapy should not be taken as an absolute, and may vary depending on the biological age of the patient.

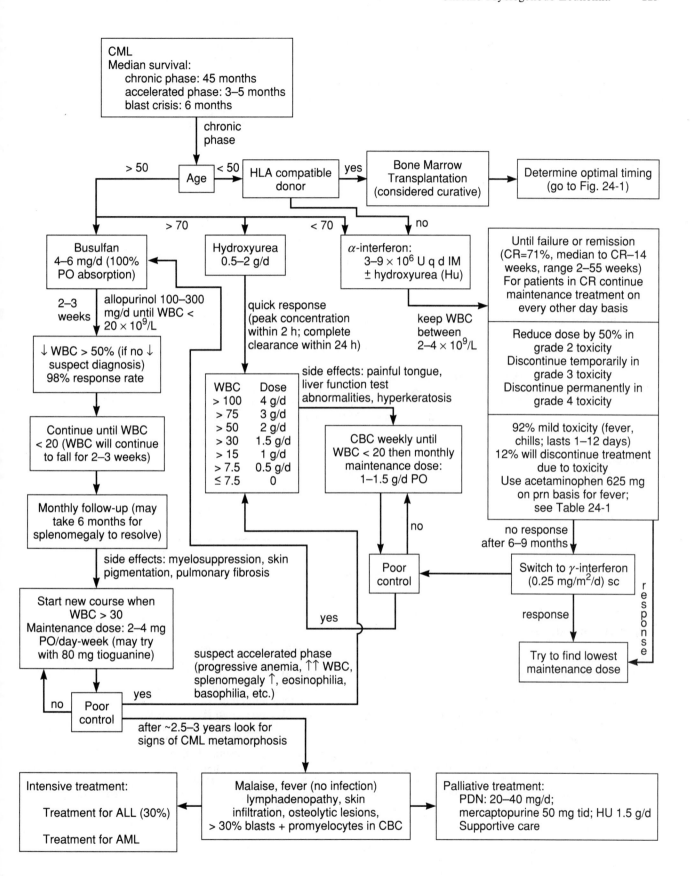

Table 24-1. Toxicity Criteria for Therapy With Interferon

Toxicity	1	2	3	4
Fever, chills, influenzalike symptoms; bone and muscle aches	Self-limiting, no therapy needed	Require antipyretics or antiinflammatory agents	Require narcotics and/or hospitalization	Life-threatening
Fatigue, performance status (Zubrod scale)	1	2	3	4
Weight loss (percentage of body weight)	0–5	6–10	11–15	>15
Renal function (creatinine in mg/100 ml)		Up to 2.5	>2.5	
Liver function Bilirubin (mg/ 100 ml)		Up to 2.5	>2.5	
SGOT (mU/ ml)		300–600	>600	
Neurologic	Does not interfere with daily activities or require medical intervention	Moderate impairment of activities, requires medical therapy	Severe impairment of activities, requires discontinuation of interferon and medical therapy	Coma, seizures, confusion, parkinsonism, severe depression
Hematologic: Granulocyte count (per μL)		1,000–2,000	<1,000	
Platelet count (× 10^3/μL)		50–100	25–50	<25

(From Talpaz et al.: Blood 69:1280, 1987, with permission.)

Suggested Readings

Denic S, Djulbegovic B, Ridzanovic Z: Optimal timing of bone marrow transplantation in chronic myelogenous leukemia. Period Biol 91:391, 1989

Kurzrock R, Kantarjian HM, Shtalrid M, Gutterman JU, Talpaz M: Philadelphia chromosome-negative chronic myelogenous leukemia without breakpoint cluster region rearrangement: a chronic myeloid leukemia with a distinct clinical course. Blood 75:445, 1990

Shtalrid M, Talpaz M, Blick M, Romero P, Kantarjian HM, Taylor K, Trujillo J, Schachner J, Gutterman JU, Kurzrock R: Philadelphia chromosome-negative chronic myelogenous leukemia with breakpoint cluster region rearrangement: molecular analysis, clinical characteristics and response to therapy. J Clin Oncol 6:1569, 1988

Talpaz M, Kantarjian H, McCredie KB, et al.: Clinical investigation of human alpha-interferon in chronic myelogenous leukemia. Blood 69:1280, 1987

Talpaz M, Kantarjian H, Kurzrock R, Gutterman JU: Update on therapeutic options for chronic myelogenous leukemia. Semin Hematol 27:31, 1990

Talpaz M, Kantarjian H, Kurzrock R, et al.: Interferon-alpha produces sustained cytogenetic responses in chronic myelogenous leukemia. Philadelphia chromosome-positive patients. Ann Intern Med 114:532, 1991

Idiopathic Myelofibrosis/ Agnogenic Myeloid Metaplasia

25

Idiopathic myelofibrosis/agnogenic myeloid metaplasia (IMF/AMM) is a disorder involving the abnormal deposition of a collagen material in the bone marrow (some 25 different names have been proposed for disorders with a prominent myelofibrotic component). While it is a clonal disorder, fibroblasts are not derived from the abnormal hematopoietic stem cell and are reactive in nature. Together with chronic myeloid leukemia (CML), essential thrombocythemia (ET), and P. Vera, it is classified as a *myeloproliferative syndrome* (MPS) (the acute form of IMF resembles acute leukemia, and will not be considered here). Aside from MPS, hairy cell leukemia should be considered in differential diagnoses as well. IMF/AMM usually affects people between 50–70 years of age and is slightly more common in males than females. Diagnostic features of IMF/ AMM are similar to other MPS disorders, as is the diagnostic workup (see Fig. 21-8 for diagnostic workup). Tests with the highest diagnostic values in IMF/AMM are *leukoerythroblastic blood picture* (combination of myeloid precursors with red blood cell (RBC) precursors, seen in virtually all patients at diagnosis; S = 100%), *splenomegaly* (S = 95–100%), and *marrow fibrosis* on bone marrow biopsy/ aspiration. Therefore, a *production rule* may be defined: *If* myeloid and erythrocyte precursors are present in the peripheral smear of a patient with splenomegaly, *then* suspect myelofibrosis (and perform bone marrow aspirate biopsy).

The course of disease varies; some patients may do well for years and not require treatment, but symptomatic patients will require treatment. Leading causes of death are infections (pneumonia being the most common), cardiac failure, thrombosis, and bleeding. Since massive splenomegaly is a characteristic feature of this disease, quite a few patients will require a splenectomy at some point during the course of the disease (for pain, hemolysis, thrombocytopenia, or portal hypertension). In experienced hands the mortality should be less than 10%, but it can vary between 7–42%.

Since there is no single randomized trial evaluating different forms of therapy, treatment decisions are based upon retrospective and individual estimates regarding the benefit/risk of different forms of therapy. Figure 25-1 outlines details of the clinical management of IMF/AMM. The median survival of patients with IMF/AMM is about 5 years, with a range of 1–15 years. Prognostic factors vary among different studies; some of them are shown in Figure 25-1. In a recent study by Demory, et al., abnormalities in karyotype (usually 20q− and 13q− deletion or additional chromosome 8) and age are the only independent prognostic factors. Therefore, a routine cytogenetic study is probably indicated in all patients with IMF/AMM, which will detect abnormalities in about 50% of cases.

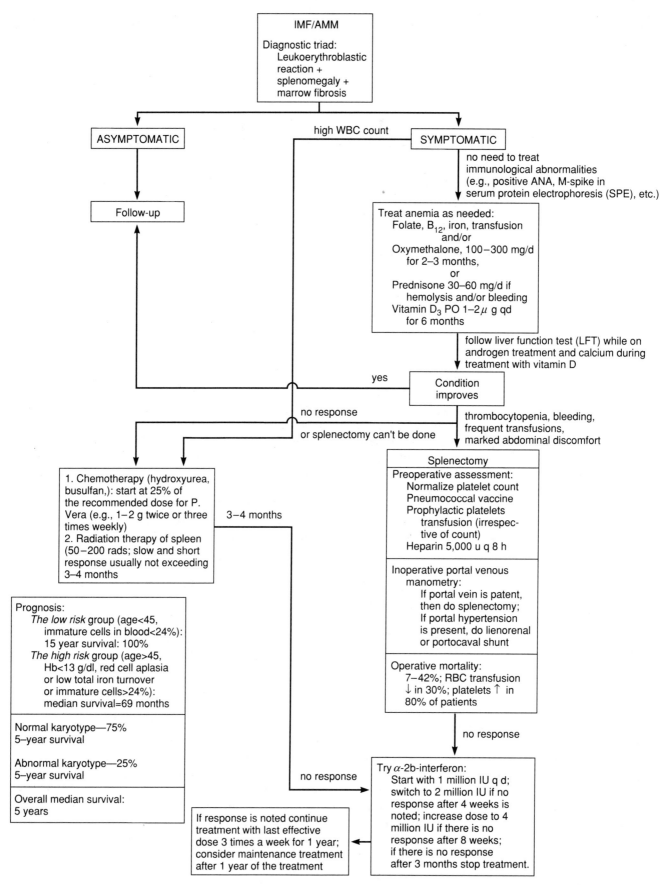

Fig. 25-1. The treatment of chronic idiopathic myelofibrosis (IMF). The construction of the algorithm is based upon the *risk/benefit estimate* and *probability of the response* to various therapeutic options available for the disease with a highly variable clinical course. Note that prognostic factors as yet do not allow us to tailor the therapy.

Suggested Readings

Barosi G, Berzuini C, Liberato LN, et al.: A prognostic classification of myelofibrosis with myeloid metaplasia. Br J Haematol 70:397, 1988

Buyssens N, Bourgeois NH: Chronic myelocytic leukemia versus idiopathic myelofibrosis. Cancer 40:1548, 1977

Demory JL, Dupriez B, Fenaux P, et al.: Cytogenic studies and their prognostic significance in agnogenic myeloid metaplasia: a report on 47 cases. Blood 72:855, 1988

Dupriez B, Demory JL, Fenaux P, Bauters F: Prognostic classification of myelofibrosis with myeloid metaplasia. Br J Haematol 71:136, 1989

Lazzarino M, Vitale AM, Gagliardi A, et al.: Interferon alpha-2b as treatment for Philadelphia-negative chronic myeloproliferative disorders with excessive thrombocytosis. Br J Haematol 72:173, 1989

Manoharan A. Treatment of myelofibrosis with hydroxyurea. Blood 76:299a, 1990

Smith RE, Chelmowski MK, Szabo EJ: Myelofibrosis: a concise review of clinical and pathologic features and treatment. Am J Hematol 29:174, 1988.

26 Chronic Lymphocytic Leukemia

Chronic lymphocytic leukemia (CLL) is the most common type of leukemia, with an age-adjusted incidence of 5.2 per 100,000 in the 55–59 age range and 30.4 per 100,000 in the 80–84 age range. This is a disease predominantly of the older population, with a median age of onset in the seventh decade. It is seen in less than 10% of people younger than age 40. The incidence in men is about twice that in women.

Phenotypically, CLL is a B-cell disease in more than 95% of all cases. Monoclonality is proven by the presence of either kappa (κ) or lambda (λ) light chains on the cell surface. A unique feature of CLL is the presence of the CD5 antigen. Some investigators feel that if CD5 is not found on cells, a diagnosis of CLL should be questioned (sensitivity of test close to 100%).

There is a strong correlation between tumor burdens as measured by the stage of disease and survival. Other factors, such as lymphocyte doubling time, pattern of bone marrow infiltration, and chromosome abnormalities are of strong prognostic significance as well. Two staging systems are currently is use: Rai's system, derived from retrospective data; and Binnet's system, derived from prospective data. The overall median survival for CLL is 4–5 years, but can vary from more than 10 years for stage 0 or A to less than 30 months for stage IV or C, retrospectively. More than 50% of patients are in the low disease stage at presentation, and therefore the key question is *whether* and *when* a patient with CLL should be treated. Studies have not shown a survival advantage from the treatment of patients with low stage (A or 0,I) over observation alone. These patients should be carefully monitored *only*. Patients with an intermediate stage of disease (B, II) should probably be treated with chlorambucil alone. More aggressive treatment (such as "little CHOP") is needed for an advanced stage of the disease (C, III/IV). One has to admit, however, that the overall response rate in CLL to chemotherapy has not been great. True complete remissions (CR) are in a range between 20–25% at best. Partial remission may be achieved in an additional 30–35% of patients. However, new chemotherapy agents are on the horizon and appear promising. Initial studies suggest that the response rate for one such agent—fludarabine—may be as high as 80% for previously untreated patients, and more than 50% for pentostatin. Third-phase trials are currently underway to evaluate the efficacy of these agents *vs* standard treatment.

Beside treatment of the disease, it is very important to treat its complications, such as infections, hemolytic anemia, and thrombocytopenia. These patients frequently have hypogammaglobulinemia, and therefore human gamma globulin (IgG) may be indicated at 2–4 week intervals. While gamma globulin (400 mg/kg) may be indicated in patients with frequent infections, decision analysis has shown that therapy results in a gain of only 0.8 quality-adjusted days per patient per year at a cost of $6 million per quality-adjusted life-year gained—a result that does not justify a routine use of IgG. Also, high doses of IgG have not been proven to be beneficial for autoimmune complications (thrombocytopenia, hemolytic anemia). A splenectomy is another treatment option frequently considered with these patients (Fig. 26-1 for details of management of CLL).

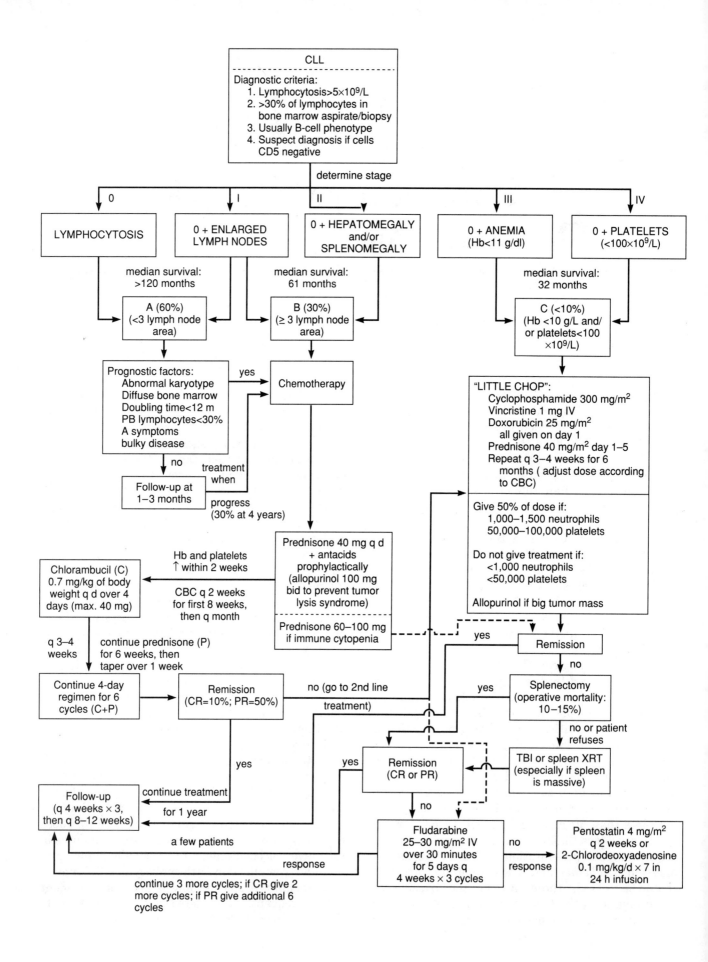

Suggested Readings

Dighiero G, Travedo P, Chevret S, et al.: B-cell chronic lymphocytic leukemia: present status and future directions. Blood 78:1901, 1991

French Cooperative Group on Chronic Lymphocytic Leukemia. Long-term results of the CHOP regimen in stage C chronic lymphocytic leukemia. Br J Haematol 73:334, 1989

French Cooperative Group on Chronic Lymphocytic Leukemia. Effects of chlorambucil and therapeutic decision in initial forms of chronic lymphocytic leukemia (Stage A): results of a randomized clinical trial on 612 patients. Blood 75:1414, 1990

French Cooperative Group on Chronic Lymphocytic Leukemia. A randomized clinical trial of chlorambucil versus COP in stage B chronic lymphocytic leukemia. Blood 75:1422, 1990

Foon KA, Rai KR, Gale PR: Chronic lymphocytic leukemia: new insights into biology and therapy. Ann Intern Med 113:525, 1990

International Workshop on Chronic Lymphocytic Leukemia. Chronic Lymphocytic leukemia: recommendations for diagnosis, staging and response criteria. Ann Intern Med 110:236, 1989

Molica S: Progression and survival in early chronic lymphocytic leukemia. Blood 78:895, 1991

Weeks JC, Tierney MR, Weinstein MC: Cost-effectiveness of prophylactic intravenous immune globulin in chronic lymphocytic leukemia. N Engl J Med 325:81, 1991

Fig. 26-1. Treatment of chronic lymphocytic leukemia (CLL). Estimates of the *risk/benefit* of different treatment options dominates decision making in the treatment of CLL. Those estimates are derived from studying the natural course of the disease and from clinical trials. Two major treatment dilemmas currently remain: when to elect *not* to treat patients, and what is the second-line treatment. An evaluation of the clinical efficacy of fludarabine as a first-line treatment is currently underway. (*Abbreviations*: PB, peripheral blood; DX, diagnosis; ↑, increased; CR, complete remission; PR, partial remission; TBI, total body irradiation; XRT, x-ray therapy.) Broken arrows/lines denote alternate strategy.

27 Leukopenia

Leukopenia is usually defined as occurring when the total white cell count (WBC) is less than 3,500/mm^3. As in the case of other hematologic problems (e.g., anemia, polycythemia, leukocytosis, etc.), the most relevant clinical question relates to the possible underlying conditions causing the leukopenia. In other words, the clinician should ask whether the low WBC is due to *primary hematologic conditions* or if it reflects *other* medical conditions. The first step is to ascertain whether other cell lines are involved (*pancytopenia*), or if we are dealing with *isolated leukopenia*. A production rule developed in the workup of anemia presenting with involvement of other cell lines (see Table 3-2) can be quite successfully applied in this setting.

Clinically, *neutropenia* is the most important reason for a decrease in the WBC. Neutropenia can be virtually excluded if the total WBC is greater than 5,000/mm^3. *Lymphopenia* may have some clinical significance, while *monocytopenia, eosinopenia* and *basopenia* rarely have practical clinical significance.

The clinical approach to neutropenia involves a distinction between disorders due to *production* of neutrophils as opposed to disorders of neutrophil *distribution* and *turnover*. If one is unsure as to which mechanism is involved, a prednisone stimulation test may help distinguish between the two. The three most important clinical problems seen with neutropenia are *aplastic anemia, acute leukemia/myelodysplastic syndrome* (MDS), and *drug-induced agranulocytosis* (pure-WBC aplasia) ("diagnosis you can't afford to miss"). Clinical information of the utmost significance includes a positive history of drug usage, which may cause neutropenia (the list is quite long, but anticancer drugs, sulfonamides, chloramphenicol, and antithyroid drugs are the first to ask

Common Drugs Causing Neutropenia

Dose-related Mechanism:
  Most chemotherapeutic agents
  (*Alkylating agents*: melphalan, cyclophosphamide, etc.
  antimetabolites: ara-C, 5-FU, 6-MP, etc.
  antitumor antibiotics: doxorubicin, etc.
  vinca alkaloids: vincristine, etc.)
  Chloramphenicol
  Ethanol
  Rifampin

Idiosyncratic:
(Usually occurs after at least a 2 week period of exposure to the drug; if it has not occurred after 3 months it will likely not occur at all.)
  Chlorpromazine and other *phenothiazines*
  Imipramine
  Antithyroid agents

  Antibiotics:
  Chloramphenicol
  Sulfonamides
  Carbenicillin
  Isoniazid
  β-lactam antibiotics

  Antihistamines:
  Phenylbutazone
  Penicillamine

Immunemediated Reactions:
  Sulfonamides
  Ampicillin
  Penicillin
  Quinidine
  Procainamide
  Thiazide and ethacrynic acid diuretics
  Allopurinol
  Cimetidine
  Gentamicin
  Nitrofurantoin

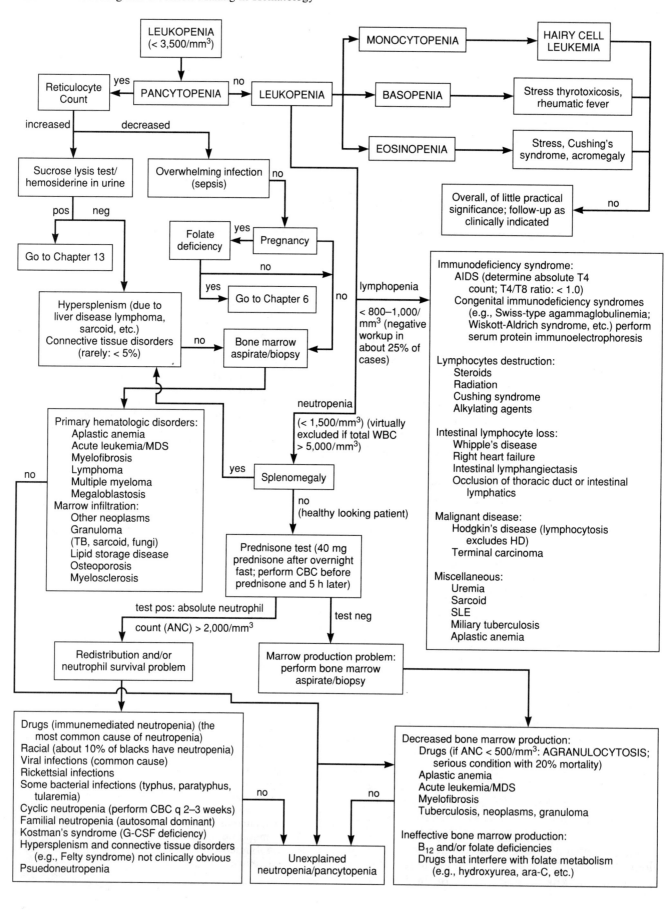

about). There are three general mechanisms by which drugs can cause neutropenia: dose-related, idiosyncratic, and immunemediated mechanism (see p. 125) for the most common drugs implicated in the cause of leukopenia). The most important physical sign one should look for is the presence of *splenomegaly/lymphadenopathy*. A bone marrow aspirate/biopsy is the diagnostic procedure with the highest yield in leukopenia caused by production disorders.

Suggested Readings

Dale DC, Hammond WP: Cyclical neutropenia: a clinical review. Blood Rev 2:1, 1988

The International Agranulocytosis and Aplastic Anemia Study. Risks of agranulocytosis and aplastic anemia. JAMA 256:1749, 1986

Mammus SW, Burton JD, Groat JD, et al.: Ibuprofen-associated pure white-cell aplasia. N Engl J Med 314:624, 1986

Ruttiman S, Clemencon D, Dubach UC: Usefulness of complete blood count as a case-finding tool in medical outpatients. Ann Intern Med 116:44, 1992

Sears D, Kickler TS, Johnson RJ, Ness PM: The diagnostic usefulness of measuring antineutrophil antibodies in neutropenic patients. Acta Hematol 76:65, 1986

Shapiro MF, Greenfield S: The complete blood count and leukocyte differential count. An approach to their rational application. Ann Intern Med 106:65, 1987

van der Veen JPW, Hack CE, Engelfriet CP, et al.: Chronic idiopathic and secondary neutropenia: clinical and serological investigations. Br J Haematol 63:161, 1986

Fig. 27-1. Algorithm for workup of leukopenia (pancytopenia). Essentially, the algorithm is based on the *physiologic reasoning* that leukopenia can occur either due to failure of marrow *production* or due to problems of *distribution* and *turnover* (see also production rule in Table 3-2). The bone marrow aspirate/biopsy is the diagnostic procedure with the highest yield in the clinical workup of leukopenia. Some authors advocate a prednisone test in order to avoid unnecessary invasive procedures. Note, however, that the sensitivity and specificity of this test is unknown (although the authors themselves use it in healthy looking patients).

28 | Myelodysplastic Syndromes

The *myelodysplastic syndromes* (MDS) are a group of clonal, heterogeneous disorders with a somewhat greater incidence than acute leukemia (3–5 per 100,000 population), occurring more frequently in the elderly male population (older than 60 years). The French-American-British Cooperative Group defined a set of production rules upon which a classification scheme was built to include the following entities: refractory anemia (RA), refractory anemia with ringed sideroblasts (RARS), chronic myelomonocytic leukemia (CMML), refractory anemia with excess blasts (RAEB), and refractory anemia with excess blasts in transformation (RAEB-T) (see Fig. 21-7). Typically, these patients will present with *mono-* (anemia, leukopenia, or thrombocytopenia) or *pancytopenia* and *hyperplastic bone marrow with dysmyelopoietic changes* (dyserythropoiesis, dysgranulopoiesis, or dysmegakaryocytopoiesis). (Hypoplastic MDS is rather rare, and before it is diagnosed it should be carefully distinguished from aplastic anemia; on the other hand, hyperplastic bone marrow with increased megakaryocytes has been misdiagnosed as ITP.) The prognosis of MDS depends on its rate of transformation to acute myeloid leukemia (AML), and typically is 10–20% for RA and RARS, 20–30% for CMML, 40–50% for RAEB, and 60–75% for RAEB-T. A median survival for RA and RARS is between 2–4 years, 18 months for CMML, and a year or less for RAEB and RAEB-T. However, more common than transformation to AML is death due to infections—between 60–70%. Ten percent of patients do survive longer than 5 years.

The standard therapy for MDS is supportive care. A selected group of younger patients with suitable HLA-compatible donors may be candidates for bone marrow transplantation (BMT). Hormonal therapy with corticosteroids and androgens has been largely unsuccessful. Steroids may, in fact, increase the risk for fatal infections, and are generally considered contraindicated in an MDS setting. Differentiation agents, such as low-dose cytosine arabinoside (ara-C), vitamin D_3, or retinoic acid have produced mixed results and are, overall, not very effective. A new and promising line of therapy may lie in the use of hematopoietic growth factors (GM-CSF, G-CSF, M-CSF, interleukin-1 and -3, and erythropoietin) in the treatment of these disorders. While there is some evidence that these agents may stimulate hematopoietic differentiation, much concern has been expressed over the possibility of accelerating the growth of a leukemic clone in patients with MDS. Some studies suggest that this may not be the case if the number of blasts in the marrow is less than 14%. Also, there is an impression that erythropoietin may be of use in the treatment of RA and RARS.

A critical element in treatment decisions is the use of *aggressive treatment vs follow-up and supportive care only*. It is recommended that this decision be based upon clinical observation of disease activity (stable *vs* progressing disease) and prognostic factors. Several scoring systems have been devised to assist in the prediction of the course of disease (see p. 131). These systems should be used in the context of other prognostic information, particularly chromosome analysis. By and large, the presence of chro-

129

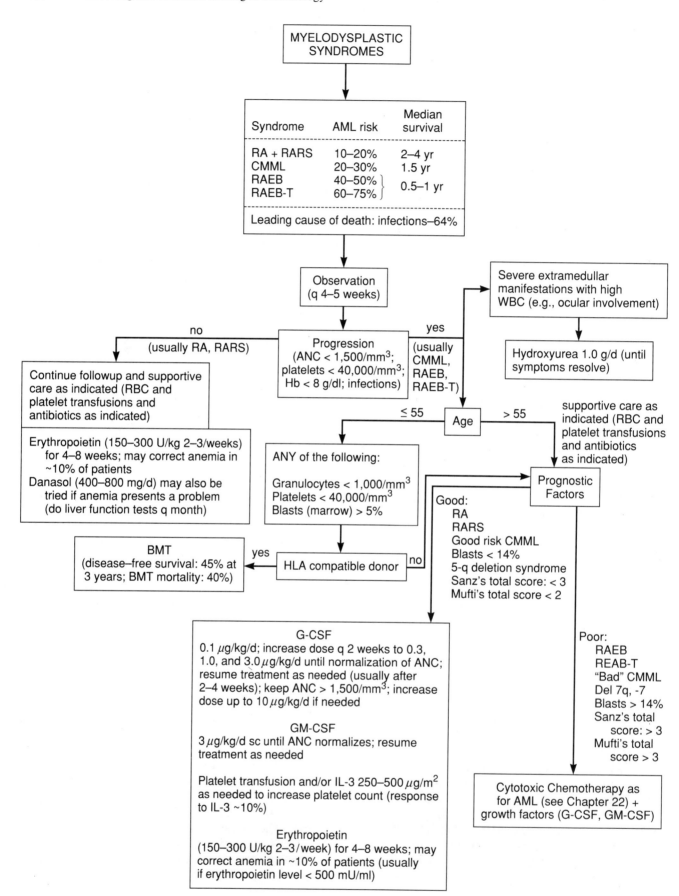

Scoring Systems for Survival Prediction in
Myelodysplastic Syndromes

Continuous Model:

Hazard rate (HR) = $\ln[h(t)/h_0(t)]$ = 0.055 (total blasts in BM)—0.0017 (platelets–173) + .022 (age–68)

If HR <.8, median survival is ≤6 months.

Simplified Categorized Model:

Parameters	Codes
Blasts in marrow <5%	0
Blasts in marrow >5 ≤ 10	1
Blasts in marrow ≥10	2
Platelet count ≥100.000/mm³	0
Platelet count >50 ≤ 100	1
Platelet count ≤50	2
Age ≤60	0
Age >60	1

If total score ≥4, then median survival ≤6 months.[a]

Parameters	Codes
Blasts in marrow ≥5%	1
Hemoglobin ≤10 g/dl	1
Neutrophil count ≤2.500/mm³	1
Platelet count ≤100.000/mm³	1

If total score is 0 or 1, median survival is 62 months (A).

If total score is 3 or 2, median survival is 22 months (B).

If total score is 4, median survival is 8.5 months (C).[b]

[a] (Data from Sanz et al. (SSS): Blood 74:395, 1989.)

[b] (Data from Mufti et al.: Br J Haematol 59:425, 1985.)

mosomal abnormalities carries a poor prognosis, but 5 q − deletion is characterized by an indolent course. Figure 28-1 shows recommended treatment decisions based upon current available information on the course of MDS and the efficacy of available treatment (strategy based upon risk/benefit estimates).

Suggested Readings

Appelbaum FR, Barrall J, Storb R, et al.: Bone marrow transplantation for patients with myelodysplasia. Pretreatment variables and outcome. Ann Intern Med 112:590, 1990

Bennett JM, Catovsky D, Daniel MT, et al.: Proposals for the classification of the myelodysplastic syndromes. Br J Haematol 51:189, 1982

Cheson BD: The myelodysplastic syndromes: current approaches to therapy. Ann Intern Med 112:932, 1990

List AF, Garewal HS, Sandberg AA: The myelodysplastic syndromes: biology and implications for management. J Clin Oncol 8:1424, 1990

Negrin RS, Haeuber DH, Nagler A, et al.: Maintenance treatment of patients with myelodysplastic syndromes using recombinant human granulocyte colony-stimulating factor. Blood 76:36, 1990

Sanz GF, San MA, Vallespi T, et al.: Two regression models and a scoring system for predicting survival and planning treatment in myelodysplastic syndromes: a multivariate analysis of prognostic factors in 370 patients. Blood 74:395, 1989

Fig. 28-1. Treatment of myelodysplastic syndromes. This strategy is based upon *benefit/risk estimates,* which in turn are derived from prognostic information on the disease course and efficacy/risk of the available treatment. Note that the clinical significance of growth factors used in this and other conditions is currently a very active area of investigation; their exact role in this situation should be fully defined within the next 5 years.

29 | Hairy Cell Leukemia

Hairy cell leukemia (HCL) is a rare disorder. It comprises about 2% of all adult leukemias and typically occurs in males (4:1; median age is about 50 years) with pancytopenia and/or monocytopenia, splenomegaly (in more than 90% of patients) and positive cytochemical staining for tartarat-resistant acid phosphatase. A bone marrow biopsy is the most reliable procedure (aspirate is typically "empty") to confirm a diagnosis of HCL, demonstrating in virtually *all* patients either diffuse or patchy infiltrates of leukemic cells.

The course of this disease varies widely. The median survival for all patients is 4 years; however, some patients may live longer than 25 years, while others die within a few months of diagnosis. As in all other hematologic malignancies, infection is the major cause of death. In addition to infections with gram-positive and gram-negative bacterias, the clinician should be aware of infections with (atypical) mycobacterium. Persistent, intermittent fevers and night sweats without an obvious source should make one suspicious of disseminated mycobacterial disease.

The major problem in the management of HCL patients is identifying those who should be treated immediately from those who can be monitored or treated by a splenectomy alone. If the marrow is *not* heavily infiltrated and the patient does *not* have pancytopenia in the absence of splenomegaly, treatment is probably not indicated. A splenectomy will be the treatment of choice in patients with massive splenomegaly or splenic rupture. All other patients should be treated by systemic therapy.

In the nineties it appears that the main problem is not the *lack* of appropriate treatment armamentarium but *which one* to choose. Only recently, in the last 5–6 years, has it been shown that several drugs are highly successful in the treatment of HCL. Interferon was the first to be shown effective controlling the disease in a substantial number of patients, inducing complete remission (CR) in 5%, normalization of the CBC in an additional 75% of patients, and a minor response in a further 14% of patients. Subsequently, it has been shown that pentostatin (deoxycoformacin) is a highly effective therapy in this disease as well, inducing CR in 59% of patients and partial remission (PR) in an additional 37%. A new report in 1990 described CR in 11 out of 12 patients treated with a *single* course of 2-chlorodeoxyadenosine. Since no comparison has been made among these agents in a single, prospective trial, it is difficult at this time to recommend the best treatment strategy, but low toxicity and a high response rate suggest that 2-chlorodeoxyadenosine may well be the drug of choice in the treatment of HCL. Prospective trials are under way to answer these questions. Until this information becomes available, Figure 29-1 may serve as a guideline to the management of patients with HCL. Note that the high cost (pentostatin) and commercial unavailability of 2-chlorodeoxyadenosine dictates the current approach to the treatment of HCL.

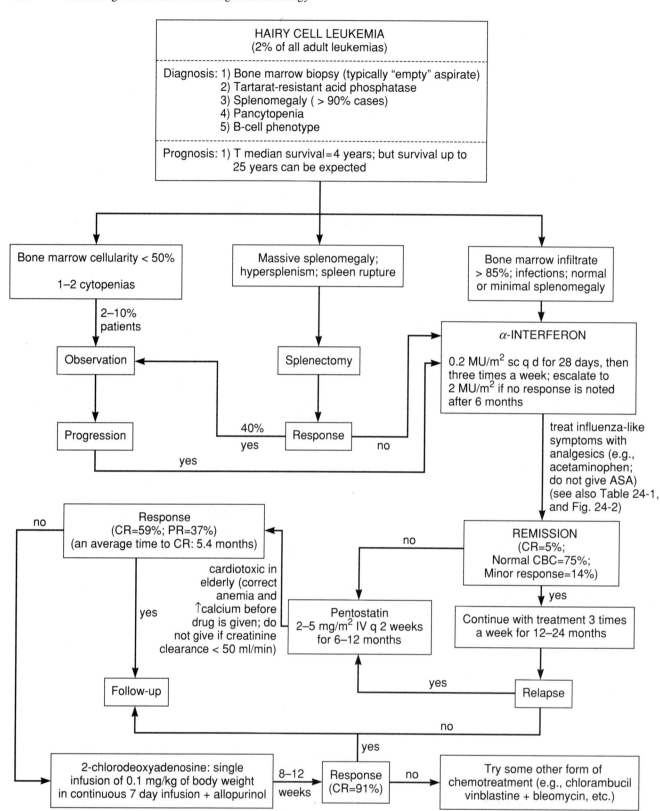

Fig. 29-1. Treatment of hairy cell leukemia. The recommended strategy is not based on the estimated efficacy of treatment but on the availability and cost of current medications (*limited resources approach*) Note that 2-chlorodeoxyadenosine is not commercially available, and pentostatin is very costly and also not readily available.

Suggested Readings

Cheson BD, Martin A: Clinical trials in hairy cell leukemia. Current status and future directions. Ann Intern Med 106:871, 1987

Golomb H, Ratain MJ: Recent advances in the treatment of hairy cell leukemia. N Engl J Med 316:870, 1987

Golomb H, Ratain MJ, Moormeier J: What is the choice of treatment for hairy cell leukemia. J Clin Oncol 7:156, 1989

Kraut EC, Bouroncle BA, Grever MR: Pentostatin in the treatment of advanced hairy cell leukemia. J Clin Oncol 7:168, 1989

Piro DL, Carrera CJ, Carson DA, Beutler E: Lasting remissions in hairy cell leukemia induced by a single infusion of 2-chlordeoxyadenosine. N Engl J Med 322:1117, 1990

Smalley RV, Anderson SA, Tuttle RL, et al.: A randomized comparison of two doses of human lymphoblastoid interferon-alpha in hairy cell leukemia. Blood 78:3133, 1991

Treatment of Immunocompromised (Neutropenic) Patients

30

Many hematologic diseases (e.g., aplastic anemia, leukemias, lymphomas, etc.) are associated with various immunologic defects. In general, these defects are related to: (1) neutropenia, (2) T cell dysfunction (cellular immunity), and (3) B cell dysfunction (humoral immunity) (see box below). In addition, other factors—such as disruption of mucosal and cutaneous barriers—contribute to and invariably lead to infection.

Neutrophils are one of the most important defenses against infection. Consequently, neutropenia caused by chemotherapy or infiltrative marrow processes has significant clinical consequences. Neutropenia is defined as an absolute neutrophil count (ANC) of less than 1,000/mm^3. The incidence of infection in neutropenic patients increases with the *duration* (100% incidence with >3 weeks neutropenia) and *severity* of neutropenia (>90% incidence with ANC<100, 50% with ANC<500/mm^3).

Infection during chemotherapy-induced neutropenia is the leading cause of death in these immunocompromised patients. In only 40% of febrile neutropenic patients can infection be documented with a positive blood culture, but if left untreated, these infections are rapidly fatal in more than 90% of cases. Similarly, waiting for the results of cultures to direct therapy will result in more deaths than empirical treatment. Thus, the basis for the clinical approach in these cases is: *begin empiric treatment in every febrile neutropenic patient.* [Fever is defined as an oral temperature of 38 C° on two occasions in 24 hours or 38.5°C on one occasion, in the absence of an obvious noninfectious cause of fever (e.g., blood transfusion).] The reasoning strategy is, in fact,

based on the high probability of death in the absence of therapy ("diagnosis you can't afford to miss"). Neutropenia without fever is not an indication for therapy.

The next important clinical decision relates to the choice of antibiotic therapy. Trials of one, two, or three antibiotic agents show comparable efficacy and toxicity. The choice of empiric therapy should be tailored to fit with local patterns of antibiotic re-

---

Immunologic Defects and Associated Pathogens

T cell Dysfunction
Gram-negative Bacilli—*Salmonella, Legionella*
Gram-positive Bacilli—*Listeria, Nocardia*
Mycobacteria—TB, avium intracellulare, kansasii
Fungi—*Cryptococcus, Candida, Histoplasma, Coccidium*
Viruses—*herpes simplex*, varicella zoster
Protozoa—*Pneumocystis, Toxoplasma, Cryptosporidium*
Helminth—*Strongyloides stercoralis*

B cell Dysfunction
Gram-negative Bacilli—*Hemophilus influenza*
Gram-positive Cocci—*Streptococcus pneumoniae*
Gram-negative Cocci—N. meningitides

Granulocytopenia
Gram-negative Bacilli—*E. coli, Klebsiella, Pseudomonas*
Gram-positive Cocci—*S. epidermis* and *aureus*
Gram-positive Bacilli—*Bacillus spp. JK Corynebacterium, Clostridium*
Fungi—*Aspergillus fumigatus* and *flavus*

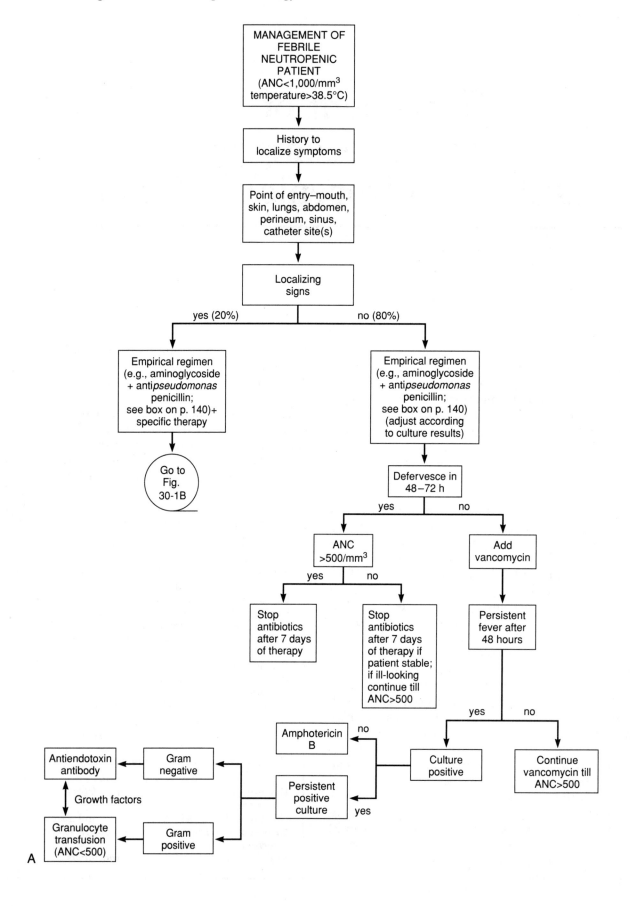

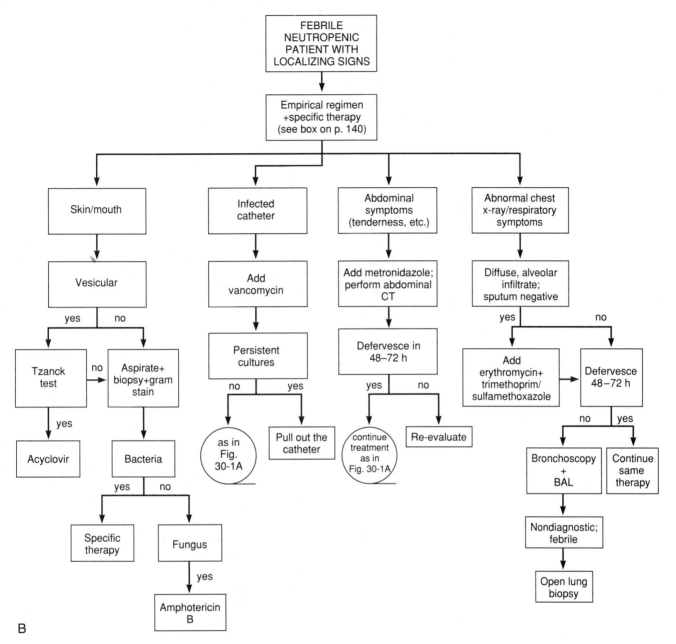

Fig. 30-1 (A and B). Treatment of febrile neutropenic patient. Reasoning strategy is highly *probabilistic,* based upon the premise that early demise (sepsis) will follow if empirical treatment is not started urgently (*"diagnosis you can't afford to miss"*). Sequential choice of therapies is also based upon estimates of the likelihood that a specific etiologic agent caused the infection in question. For example, the initial treatment is targeted against bacterial agents, first to cover a broad spectrum of gram-positive and gram-negative bacteria (especially *Pseudomonas aeruginosa*), then against gram-positive bacteria such as *Staphylococcus* (vancomycin added), then to cover fungi, as the likelihood of these infections increases with the duration of neutropenia. Obviously, this empirical (probabilistic) strategy will be modified as specific agents are isolated or a particular set of symptoms suggests a likely pathogen (Fig. 30-1B). (BAL–bronchoalveolar lavage.)

Antibiotics in Treatment of Neutropenic Patient

1. Empiric therapy:
   Amikacin 5 mg/kg IV every 8 hrs
      and
   Piperacillin 3 g IV every 6 hrs or equivalent regimen (adjust for renal or hepatic dysfunction) Peak and trough levels of Amikacin must be checked with the fourth dose. Antibiotics must be modified based on culture results.

2. Vancomycin 1 g IV every 12 hrs given as 1 hour infusion. Check peak and trough levels as indicated.

3. Acyclovir 250 mg/m^2 IV over 1 hr every 8 hrs × 7 days.

4. Amphotericin 1 mg IV in 50 cc 5% dextrose over 10 minutes. Check blood pressure, pulse, and respiration every 10 min (test dose). If no reaction or chills and fever only, 0.5–1 mg/kg IV over 1–3 hrs. Premedicate with acetaminophen (Tylenol) 650 mg PO, Benadryl 25 mg IV, Demerol 50 mg IV and PRN chills. Hydrocortisone 50 mg may be added. Potassium, magnesium, and creatinine must be monitored. If fungus identified, continue till 1–2 g total dose.

5. Metronidazole (Flagyl) 15 mg/kg IV, then 7.5 mg/kg every 6 hrs.

6. G-CSF/GM-CSF 250 μg/m^2 subcutaneously × 7–14 days.

7. Granulocyte Transfusions: >10^{10} cells from related donor daily × 4–9 days. Premedicate with Tylenol orally, Benadryl 25–50 mg IV and hydrocortisone 100 mg IV. Use blood filter and monitor vital signs.

8. Trimethoprim-Sulfamethoxazole 5 mg/kg IV every 6 hrs × 2–3 wks.

General Measures in Treatment of Granulocytopenia

1. Avoid fresh fruits, fresh vegetables, and black pepper (may contain gram-negative bacteria and fungi).

2. Avoid fresh flowers (may contain fungi).

3. Check water supply and avoid humidifiers (*Legionella*).

4. Careful mouth, dental, and venous access device care. One protocol for mouth care: (1) peridex 10 ml swish and spit; (2) baking soda swish and spit; (3) clotrimazole troche 10 ml dissolved in mouth, or amphotericin B oral solution (25 mg/250 ml of sterile water) 15 ml swish and swallow. Perform mouth care 6 times a day.

5. Stool softeners and a high-fiber diet.

6. Selective microbial prophylaxis: trimethoprim-sulfamethoxazole DS 1 PO bid 2–3/week (high-dose therapy/T cell dysfunction).

7. Strict hand-washing by personnel and visitors.

8. Prophylactic Ciprofloxacin 500 mg every 12 hrs (AML/ALL induction) (preliminary data).

sistance. Overall, a combination of an aminoglycoside with a beta-lactam agent is still preferred by the majority of physicians (see box opposite).

Bacterial pathogens are the major culprits in infection in immunocompromised patients. In the last decade the spectrum of bacterial infections has changed from predominantly gram-negative organisms to gram-positive organisms (gram-positive isolated >50% of the time). The incidence of fungal infection is 5%, but increases as the duration of neutropenia increases, especially in the face of broad spectrum antibiotic therapy (30% incidence after 7 days of ANC<500/mm^3). Fungal infections have a 70–80% mortality rate with long-standing neutropenia, despite amphotericin B. Treatment strategies for neutropenic patients must take into account the expected duration of neutropenia.

Ancillary measures—such as hand-washing—are usually used, since nearly half the infections are caused by organisms acquired in hospitals (see second box). Since more than 80% of infections in the neutropenic patient can be traced to host endogenous flora, the need for routine sterilization of these areas is being evaluated. In patients who are expected to have prolonged neutropenia, surveillance cultures of nares, throat, perianal area, and stool for bacteria, fungus, and virus may facilitate the choice of empiric therapy. The surveillance cultures may be helpful for those patients who become febrile and initially defervesce, since nearly 40% of them will become febrile again. Preliminary studies evaluating the efficacy of prophylactic therapy with fluorinated quinolones in neutropenic patients with hematologic malignancies are promising.

The clinical use of hematopoietic growth factors such as granulocyte colony-stimulating factor (G-CSF) and granulocyte-macrophage colony-stimulating factor (GM-CSF) have been shown to decrease the incidence of infection and length of hospitalization associated with chemotherapy. Macrophage colony-stimulating factor (M-CSF) is being evaluated as an adjunct to amphotericin B in immunocompromised patients with fungal infections. Figure 30-1 shows algorithms for treatment of febrile neutropenic patients. The second box in this chapter shows dosages and other details of management of patients with granulocytopenia.

Suggested Readings

Buckner CD, Clift RA: Prophylaxis and treatment of infection of the immunocompromised host by granulocyte transfusions. Clin Hematol 13:557, 1984

The GIMEMA Infection Program. Prevention of bacterial infection in neutropenic patients with hematologic malignancies. Ann Intern Med 115:7, 1991

Gucalp R: Management of the febrile neutropenic patient with cancer. Oncology 5:137, 1991

Hughes WT, Armstrong D, Bodey GP, et al.: Guidelines for the use of antimicrobials in neutropenic patients with unexplained fever. J Infect Dis 161:381, 1990

Pizzo PA: After empiric therapy: what to do until the granulocyte comes back. Rev Infect Dis 9:214, 1987

Walsh TJ, Schimpff SC: Infection in immunosuppressed patients. In Brain MC, Carbone PP (eds.): Current Therapy in Hematology/Oncology 3. BC Decker, Toronto, 1988

Winston DJ, Winston GH, Bruckner DA, Champlin RE: Beta-lactam antibiotic therapy in febrile granulocytopenic patients. Ann Intern Med 115:849, 1991

31 | Lymphadenopathy: Diagnostic Approach

Initial reasoning elements in the diagnostic workup of the patient with enlarged *lymphadenopathy* involves the application of *causal reasoning* (a distinction between *localized vs generalized* adenopathy, based upon an understanding of the different etiology of isolated and generalized adenopathy) and an *availability and representative heuristic* (through ordering readily available complete blood count (CBC) with differential count—see Chapter 1). A complete CBC also identifies certain conditions with high specificity, and thus is one of the most useful initial tests. It is also very sensitive for the Epstein-Barr (EB) virus infection (a common virus infection among young adults). However, its sensitivity is rather low for all varieties of other diseases, and so cannot be used for screening purposes (see Chapter 2). Numerous diagnostic hypotheses can be triggered by the application of certain clinical rules that, although not scientifically validated, have been largely incorporated into medical practice. The key element in the diagnostic workup relates to a decision as to *when* to perform a biopsy, as this is the test with the overall greatest diagnostic yield. A rule has been derived to assist in this decision in young patients. Figures 31-1A and 1B show algorithms constructed upon the principles mentioned. Overall, it can be noted that the ordering of a CBC, chest x-ray, PPD skin test, serology for EB virus, CM virus, and toxoplasmosis (i.e., six diagnostic tests only) will precede a biopsy of lymph nodes in most cases involving the workup of a patient with lymphadenopathy. This will be sufficient in the vast majority of patients. However, one also has to realize that in 40–60% of cases even a biopsy can be nondiagnostic, and

therefore the evaluation of patients with lymphadenopathy must be *individualized*. Occasionally, repeated biopsies will be necessary to reach a diagnosis. Operating test characteristics of some tests used in the evaluation of patients with lymphadenopathy are shown in Table 31-1. Some useful data and *production rules* for workup of lymphadenopathy are:

1. Any peripheral lymph node 1 cm in size or greater that does not show signs of regression after 6 weeks of observation should be biopsied. Alternatively, in young patients use the "biopsy score" rule to decide whether to perform a biopsy (see Fig. 31-1A).

2. The probability of malignancy in enlarged peripheral lymph nodes increases steadily with age: 10% of neck masses in children are malignant, compared with 80% of neck masses in adults older than 40 years.

3. A firm, nontender mass in the neck of a patient over 40 is probably metastatic cancer, while soft nodes are more likely to be either benign or lymphomas. The probability of lymphoma is much higher in the younger population than metastatic carcinoma. Enlarged supraclavicular nodes should be considered malignant until proven otherwise. In children *and* young adults with generalized adenopathy, an infectious etiology is the most common cause.

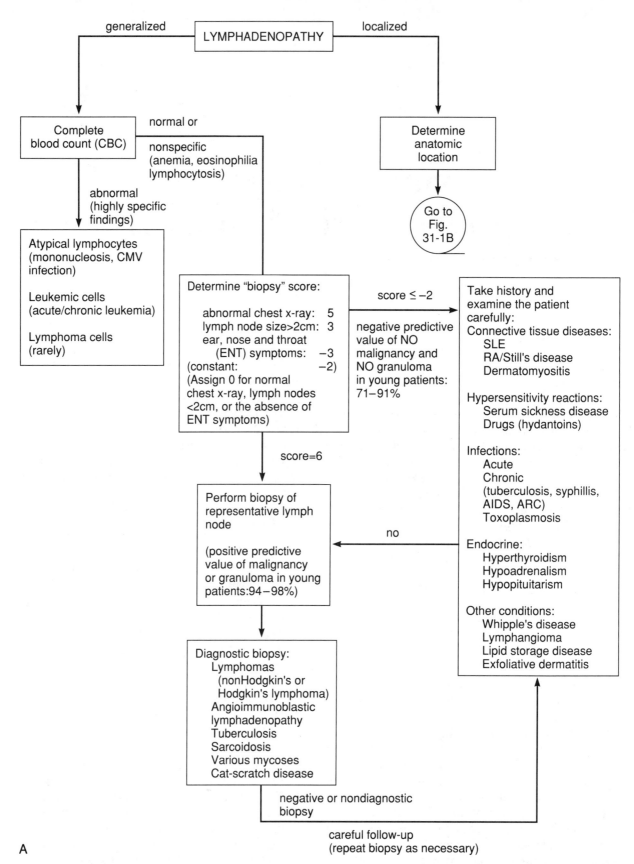

Fig. 31-1 (A and B). Diagnostic approach to lymphadenopathy. The initial approach involves a combination of *causal reasoning* (localized *vs* generalized lymphadenopathy) with an *availability and representative heuristic* approach (ordering CBC, which is also a highly specific test for certain conditions). Application of the *production rule* (any superficial lymph node 1 cm or greater that does not show signs of regression after 6 weeks of observation should be biopsied) or a statistically developed "biopsy" score dominates further clinical workup.

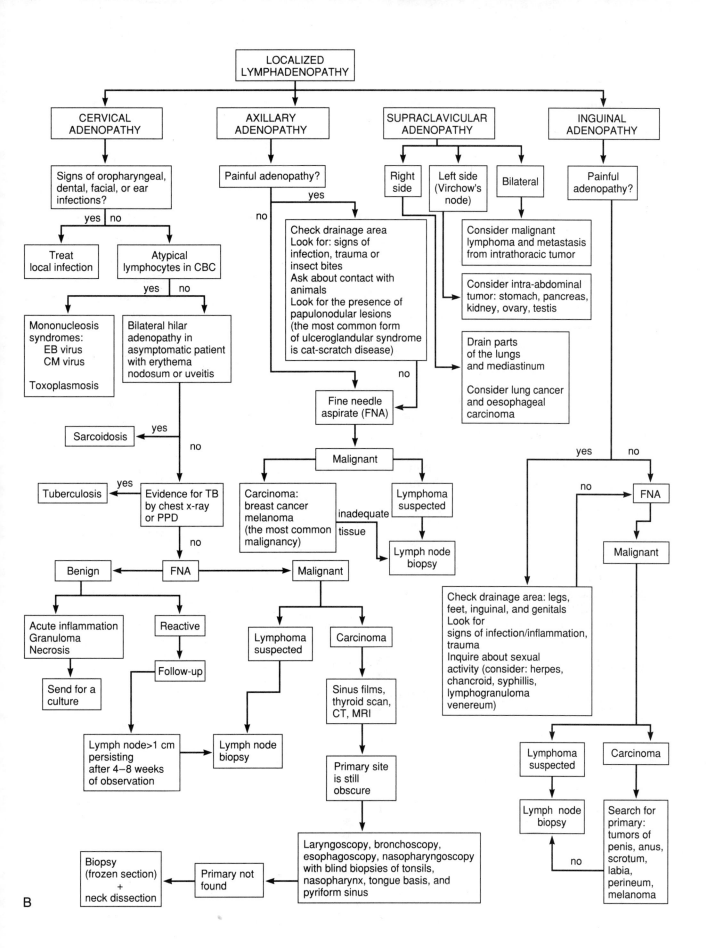

LOCALIZED LYMPHADENOPATHY

CERVICAL ADENOPATHY

Signs of oropharyngeal, dental, facial, or ear infections?

yes → Treat local infection

no → Atypical lymphocytes in CBC

yes → Mononucleosis syndromes:
EB virus
CM virus

Toxoplasmosis

no → Bilateral hilar adenopathy in asymptomatic patient with erythema nodosum or uveitis

yes → Sarcoidosis

no → Evidence for TB by chest x-ray or PPD

yes → Tuberculosis

no → FNA

Benign → Acute inflammation
Granuloma
Necrosis → Send for a culture

Reactive → Follow-up → Lymph node>1 cm persisting after 4–8 weeks of observation → Lymph node biopsy

Malignant → Lymphoma suspected → Lymph node biopsy

Malignant → Carcinoma → Sinus films, thyroid scan, CT, MRI → Primary site is still obscure → Laryngoscopy, bronchoscopy, esophagoscopy, nasopharyngoscopy with blind biopsies of tonsils, nasopharynx, tongue basis, and pyriform sinus → Primary not found → Biopsy (frozen section) + neck dissection

AXILLARY ADENOPATHY

Painful adenopathy?

yes / no → Check drainage area
Look for: signs of infection, trauma or insect bites
Ask about contact with animals
Look for the presence of papulonodular lesions (the most common form of ulceroglandular syndrome is cat-scratch disease)

→ Fine needle aspirate (FNA)

→ Malignant

Carcinoma: breast cancer melanoma (the most common malignancy)

inadequate tissue → Lymph node biopsy

Lymphoma suspected → Lymph node biopsy

SUPRACLAVICULAR ADENOPATHY

Right side / Left side (Virchow's node) / Bilateral

Consider malignant lymphoma and metastasis from intrathoracic tumor

Consider intra-abdominal tumor: stomach, pancreas, kidney, ovary, testis

Drain parts of the lungs and mediastinum

Consider lung cancer and oesophageal carcinoma

INGUINAL ADENOPATHY

Painful adenopathy?

yes / no → FNA → Malignant

Check drainage area: legs, feet, inguinal, and genitals
Look for
signs of infection/inflammation, trauma
Inquire about sexual activity (consider: herpes, chancroid, syphillis, lymphogranuloma venereum)

Lymphoma suspected → Lymph node biopsy

no

Carcinoma → Search for primary: tumors of penis, anus, scrotum, labia, perineum, melanoma

B

Table 31-1. Operating Characteristics of Some Tests Used in Evaluation of Patients With Enlarged Peripheral Lymph Nodes

Test	Sensitivity (%)	Specificity (%)	Disease
"Biopsy" score	82–96	80–100	Malignancy or granuloma (age 9–25 years)
Fine needle aspiration	93	95	TB, malignancy, sarcoid, lymphadenitis
Mantoux (+)	74	100 (?)	TB lymphadenitis
Fever, sore throat, lymphadenopathy	100	?	Infectious mononucleosis
Atypical lymphocytes (>10%)	90	98	Infectious mononucleosis
EB Virus antibody	99	100	Infectious mononucleosis
Chest X-ray: bilateral hilar adenopathy in asymptomatic patient	75	99	Sarcoidosis

4. In young adults with an acute onset of cervical adenopathy, with no signs of head and neck infections, infectious mononucleosis syndrome is the most likely diagnosis. However, if fever, sore throat, and lymphadenopathy are all absent, infection with EB can be eliminated (S = 100% for the presence of any of these signs).

5. In patients with nondiagnostic biopsy or with atypical hyperplasia of lymph nodes, there should be little hesitation in repeating the biopsy, since 25–30% of such patients will subsequently develop a disease (usually a lymphoma).

Selected Readings

Dandapat MC, Mashra BM, Dash SP, Kar PK: Peripheral lymph node tuberculosis: a review of 80 cases. Br J Surg 77:911, 1990

Hajek PC, Salomonowitz E, Turk R, Tscholakoff D, Kupman W, Czembirek H: Lymph nodes of the neck: evaluation with US. Radiology 158:739, 1986

Jacobs C: The internist in the management of head and neck cancer. Ann Int Med 113:771, 1990

Kardos TF, Maygarden SJ, Blumberg AK, et al.: Fine needle aspiration biopsy in the management of young adults with peripheral lymphadenopathy. Cancer 63:703, 1989

Kendel G, Grossman RF: Large neck node, silent chest mass. Hosp Pract 21(4):79, 1986

Libman H: Generalized lymphadenopathy. J Gen Intern Med 2:48, 1987

Premachandra DJ, McRae D, Prinsley P: Missed diagnosis: Biopsy of neck lumps in adults should be preceded by examination of the upper aerodigestive tract. Postgrad Med J 66:113, 1990

Slap GB, Brooks JSJ, Schwartz JS: When to perform biopsies of enlarged peripheral lymph nodes in young patients. JAMA 252:1321, 1984

Slap GB, Connor JL, Wigton RS, Schwartz JS: Validation of a model to identify young patients for lymph node biopsy. JAMA 255:2768, 1986

Splenomegaly as a Dominant Clinical Feature: Diagnostic Approach

32

The incidence of *splenomegaly* found during physical examination in the United States has ranged from 2–6%. Palpable spleens are not always abnormal (3–5%) and abnormal spleens are not always palpable. The most cited sensitivity and specificity of various bedside maneuvers in the detection of splenomegaly varies between about 46–79%* and 69–100%, respectively (see Table 32-1). A technetium scan is considered to be the best test for detection of an enlarged spleen, although comparable results may be achieved with ultrasound (US) and the new generation of CT scanners.

Reasoning strategies that rely upon availability and representative heuristic (through ready availability of CBC) dominate the clinical workup of a patient with an enlarged spleen. Thus, the vast majority of diagnoses can be suspected by a determination from the CBC alone. Its determination also parallels an estimate that lymphoproliferative and myeloproliferative diseases are among the most common causes of splenomegaly, and therefore represents the logical choice in a clinical workup. If a diagnostic hypothesis cannot be triggered by a CBC alone, then splenomegaly should be interpreted within the overall clinical picture. The representative heuristic and production rules development are reasoning strategies commonly employed here.

A series of *production rules* have been developed to assist in the triggering of a diagnostic hypothesis that can explain splenomegaly. Overall, the predictive values of these rules have not been validated

but, in this author's experience, have been very useful. Some of these *rules* are:

1. *If* the patient has a history of recent car accidents or trauma and spleen (mass) is palpated in left lower hypochondrium, *then* consider a splenic hematoma (rupture).
2. *If* the patient has a (chronically) enlarged spleen and enlarged lymph nodes, *then* consider lymphoma (perform biopsy) until proven otherwise.
3. In young, acutely ill patients with fever, cervical adenopathy, and sore throat, think of infectious mononucleosis.
4. In patients with erythema nodosum (particularly in young females), perform a

Table 32-1. Receiver Operating Characteristics of Physical Exam in Detection of Splenomegaly

Test	Sensitivity (%)	Specificity (%)
Splenic percussion sign	79	46
Traube's space percussion	62	72
Palpation	54–61	69–100
Percussion + palpation	46	97

---

* Some retrospective studies found sensitivity as low as 20%.

147

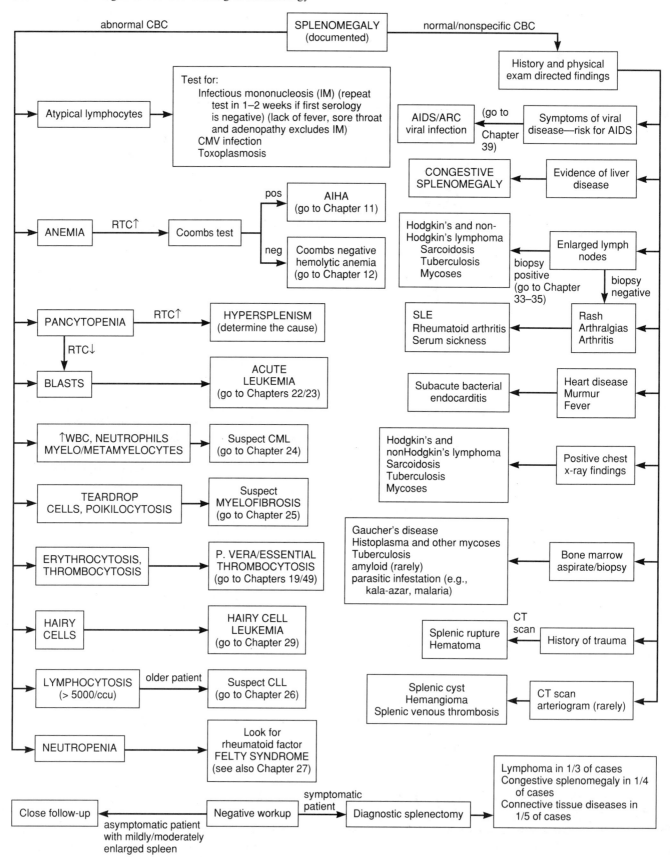

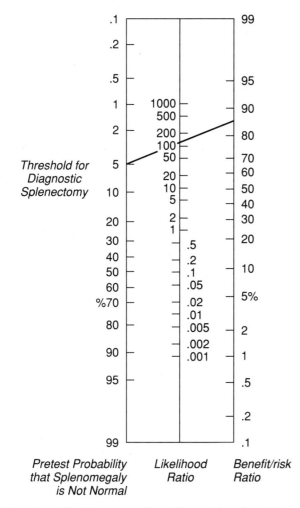

Threshold for
Diagnostic
Splenectomy

Pretest Probability
that Splenomegaly
is Not Normal

Likelihood
Ratio

Benefit/risk
Ratio

Fig. 32-2. Decision to perform diagnostic splenectomy in young, asymptomatic population. If we assume that this test (diagnostic splenectomy) will be 100% sensitive and 99% specific, and the pretest probability of not-normal etiology in the young population is not greater than 5%, then diagnostic splenectomy should be performed only if the *benefit/risk ratio* in an individual patient is greater than 80% (i.e., in a situation where clinical circumstances would likely point to possible underlying pathology—confer with Fig. 1-6).

chest x-ray (finding of bilateral hilar adenopathy is virtually a confirmation of sarcoidosis).
5. In patients with big spleen, teardrop cells, and poikilocytosis, consider myelofibrosis (perform bone marrow aspirate/biopsy).
6. In older patients with absolute lymphocytosis (>5000/μl), suspect chronic lymphatic leukemia.
7. Hypersplenism is characterized by a large spleen, pancytopenia, and active marrow ("large spleen + empty blood + full marrow").

Relatively common causes of *"asymptomatic"* splenomegaly are cirrhosis, agnogenic myeloid metaplasia, Gaucher's disease, splenic cyst, sarcoidosis, mild hereditary spherocytosis, and amyloidosis.

Spleen size is an important factor that may narrow (decrease) a number of differential diagnostic possibilities. *Marked splenomegaly* is a feature of relatively few illnesses. They include: agnogenic myeloid metaplasia (myelofibrosis), chronic myelocytic leukemia, hairy cell leukemia, and splenic lymphoma. Less common causes of marked splenomegaly are: Felty syndrome, sarcoidosis, thalassemia major, Gaucher's disease, and parasitic infection (Kala-Azar).

Overall, a CBC, liver function tests, chest x-ray, antinuclear antibody and rheumatoid factor are noninvasive tests with the greatest diagnostic yield and should be done before invasive tests are considered. The major decision in a diagnostic workup is whether and when to perform a *diagnostic splenectomy*. When the workup suggested in Figure 32-1 is negative, a diagnostic splenectomy seems to be justified in middle-aged or older symptomatic persons, where the risk of surgery does not seem to outweigh the benefit of diagnosis. In young, asymptomatic patients, the traditional recommendation would be follow-up. Decision analysis corroborates this common sense recommendation, indicating that diagnostic splenectomy should be performed only if *benefit/risk* is very high (>80%) (Figure 32-2).

Fig. 32-1. Algorithm for clinical workup of splenomegaly. This strategy is based upon the use of a readily available complete blood count (CBC) (the use of principle of availability and representative heuristic), which also detects the most common hematologic disorders. The rest of the workup is dominated by diagnostic triggering associated with a particular clinical picture (based upon *representative heuristic* and *a set of production rules*). Note that for some conditions in which splenomegaly is not a dominant clinical feature *or* a useful clue in the initial workup of a patient have been excluded from the presented algorithm.

Suggested Readings

Arkles LB, Gill GD, Molan MP: A palpable spleen is not necessarily enlarged or pathological. Med J Aust 145:15, 1986

Barkun AN, Camus M, Green L, et al.: The bedside assessment of splenic enlargement. Am J Med 91:512, 1991

Billinghurst JR: The big spleen. Br J Hosp Med 20:413, 1978

Butler JJ: Pathology of the spleen in benign and malignant conditions. Histopathology 7:453, 1983

Eichner ER, Whitfield CL: Splenomegaly. An algorithmic approach. JAMA 246:2858, 1981

Halpern S, Coel M, Ashburn W, et al.: Correlation of liver and spleen size. Determinations by nuclear medicine studies and physical exam. Arch Intern Med 134:123, 1974

King DJ, Dawson AA, Thompson WD: Splenectomy in patients with malignant lymphoma presenting with massive splenomegaly. Eur J Haematol 38:162, 1987

33 | Lymphomas: Diagnostic Workup

Malignant lymphomas include a broad spectrum of clinically and pathologically diverse neoplasms of the immune system. Hodgkin's disease (HD) and nonHodgkin's lymphoma (NHL) comprise about 1% and 3% of all cancers in the United States, respectively. Lymphomas and leukemias together account for more deaths per year than breast cancer (46,800 *vs* 44,300 in 1990). The age distribution is bimodal, with a peak incidence in adolescence and after 50 years of age. Enlarged peripheral lymph nodes are the most common presenting symptom in lymphomas (60–70%). In Hodgkin's disease, 60–80% of patients present with cervical adenopathy, 5–20% with axillary, and 6–12% with inguinal adenopathy; mediastinal involvement is present in about 60% of cases and isolated infradiaphragmatic adenopathy in only 5–10% of cases. Mesenteric involvement is rare in HD but quite common in NHL. This can be translated into a clinical production rule: *Malignant lymphomas should always be considered in a differential diagnosis of enlarged lymph nodes and splenomegaly* (see Chapters 31, 32), but also in *any* patient presenting with unexplained fever, weight loss, pruritus, or superior vena cava syndrome. The key decision is when to perform a lymph node *biopsy* (see Chapter 31); an adequate surgical biopsy is of utmost importance. Inguinal nodes should not be biopsied if equally suspicious peripheral nodes are present elsewhere. Although not a substitute for morphologic examination, use of immunohistochemistry is a useful supplement to accurate diagnosis. Interobserver concordance of diagnoses rose substantially when immunohistochemical stains were combined with hematoxylin and eosin morphologic examination.

Histopathologic Classification of Malignant Lymphomas

NonHodgkin's Lymphoma: Working Formulation—1981

Low-grade (5–10%):
    Small lymphocytic, with or without plasmacytoid differentiation
    Follicular, small cleaved
    Follicular, mixed small cleaved and large cell
Intermediate-grade (65–70%):
    Follicular, large cell
    Diffuse, small cleaved
    Diffuse, mixed, small, and large cell
    Diffuse, large cell
High-grade (20%):
    Large cell, immunoblastic
    Lymphoblastic (convoluted or nonconvoluted)
    Small noncleaved cell
Others:
    Cutaneous T cell
    Histocytic neoplasia
    Anaplastic (Ki) large cell lymphoma
    Monocytoid B cell lymphoma (low grade)
    Mantle zone (diffuse intermediate) lymphomas

Histopathologic Classification of Hodgkin's Disease

Lymphocyte Predominant (LP)	15%
Nodular Sclerosis (NS)	70%
Mixed Cellularity (MC)	10%
Lymphocyte Depleted (LP)	5%

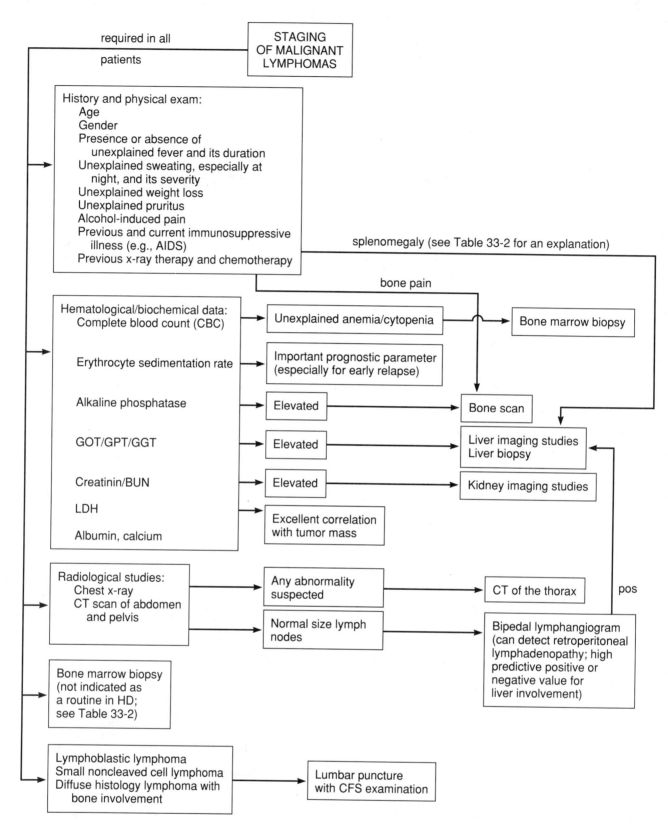

Fig. 33-1. Guidelines for staging in malignant lymphomas (see also Table 33-2 and Fig. 33-2). The goal of staging is to accurately describe the extension of disease. These guidelines are based on the Ann Arbor staging classification and its Cotswolds modification for staging in Hodgkin's disease (HD) (Tbl 33-1) Note: due to lack of general acceptance, some prognostic factors—such as copper in HD and β₂-microglobulin in NHL are not included (see also Chapter 35 on the treatment of NHL).

Table 33-1. The Ann Arbor Staging Classification Cotswolds Modifications of Hodgkin's Disease

Stage I:	Involvement of a single lymph node region (I) or single extralymphatic site (I$_E$).
Stage II:	Involvement of two or more lymph node regions on the same side of the diaphragm (II) or localized involvement of an extralymphatic site and one or more lymph node regions on the same side of the diaphragm (II$_E$).
	The number of anatomical sites involved is indicated by a suffix (e.g., II3).
Stage III$_1$:	Involvement of lymph nodes on both sides of diaphragm. Abdominal disease is limited to the upper abdomen (i.e., spleen, splenic hilar nodes, celiac nodes, porta hepatitis node).
Stage III$_2$:	Involvement of lymph nodes on both sides of diaphragm. Abdominal disease includes para-aortic, mesenteric, and iliac involvement with or without disease in the upper abdomen.
Stage IV:	Disseminated involvement of one or more extralymphatic organs or tissues with or without associated lymph node disease.

A	No symptoms
B	Fever, night sweats, or weight loss of more than 10% of body weight in the previous 6 months
X	Bulky disease (greater than 10 cm in maximum dimension; greater than ⅓ of the internal transverse diameter of the thorax at the level T5/T6)
E	Limited involvement of a single extranodal site
CS	Clinical stage: when based solely on physical examination and imaging techniques
PS	Pathologic stage: when based on biopsies

The Ann Arbor staging classification, modified from Lister et al.: J Clin Oncol 7:1630, 1989, with permission.

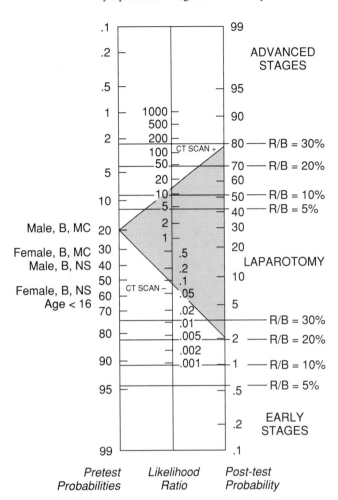

Pretest Probabilities   Likelihood Ratio   Post-test Probability

Fig. 33-2. Nomogram for determination of *probability* as to when a staging laparotomy should be performed. It is based upon a calculation of decision thresholds as discussed in Chapter I (see Fig. 1-6). In the illustrated example, testing and treatment threshold probabilities are shown after CT scan (with sensitivity and specificity to detect abdominal disease = 91%) is positive or negative, respectively. Threshold levels for four risk/benefit (R/B) ratios are shown; these are probabilities where expected treatment benefit (B) to patients with the disease equals the expected risks (R) to those without $\left(p = \dfrac{R}{B + R} \right)$.

Management action—XRT, laparotomy, chemotherapy— will depend on calculated post-test probability (i.e., whether patient is in early, "indeterminate," or advanced stage). This nomogram is particularly suitable for use with prognostic factors to estimate pretest probabilities of stage of disease. Pretest probability estimates that the patient is in an early stage of disease, as shown in the figure taken from Rutheford CJ et al: Br J Haematol 44:347, 1980. *Note:* staging is not necessary if chemotherapy will be selected as an up-front treatment.

Table 33-2. Clinical Features of Lymphoma That Are Important in Medical Decision Making

	Hodgkin's Disease (HD)	NonHodgkin's Lymphoma (NHL)	Comment
Histologic Subtype	Not as important as in NHL	Crucial	Treatment strategy in low-grade, intermediate-grade, and high-grade NHL is quite different.
Ann Arbor Staging System	Essential for planning appropriate management	Much less important in NHL than in HD	Radiation has very limited role in the primary treatment of NHL and chemotherapy is initial treatment of choice in the majority of NHL, even in early stages.
Bilateral Bone Marrow Biopsy	Bone marrow biopsies are required in patients with advanced disease, splenic involvement, and elevated serum alkaline phosphatase.	Standard workup; essential in all patients with high-grade lymphomas	Bone marrow involvement occurs in 5–20% of patients with HD and in 60–80% of patients with low-grade NHL.
Bilateral Lymphogram of Lower Extremities	Required in all patients with nodes <1.5 cm by CT (but only if XRT is considered in therapy)	Not required as a routine procedure	Overall S and Sp = 90%, comparable to CT; better than CT for para-aortic nodes (S = 82%, Sp = 100% vs S = 76% and Sp = 90%, respectively); CT better for high para-aortic nodes and mesenteric nodes
Osseous Involvement	Rare	5–15% of all patients as initial presentation	Bone scan required more often in NHL than in HD
Liver Involvement	Rare (5% of patients at diagnosis) without splenic involvement	40–60% in small lymphocytic and small cleaved cell lymphomas	Liver biopsy is rarely required (more often in NHL than in HD); dx. criteria by imaging technique: multiple focal defects that are neither cystic nor vascular noted with at least two techniques; *spleen involvement*: clearly palpable spleen or equivocal palpable spleen confirmed by radiological technique (radiological enlargement alone is not adequate).
CNS Disease	Quite rare	25% of patients with diffuse histology and bone marrow disease	Lumbar puncture is recommended in NHL patients with diffuse histology, bone marrow, testicular, or epidural tumor involvement.

Abbreviations: CT, computed tomography; XRT, x-ray therapy; CNS, central nervous system; dx, diagnostic

Once a pathologic diagnosis is made, the determination of the *histological subtype* and *tumor burden* is of critical importance in continued patient management. The box below and Table 33-1 show histopathologic classification and modified Ann Arbor staging classification of HD and NHL. Table 33-2 shows some additional clinical features of the lymphoma in terms of their importance in management decision making. Figure 33-1 shows further guidelines for accurate diagnostic staging in lymphoma patient.

Staging workup follows a physiologic line of reasoning, because of the direct relationship between prognosis and the stage of disease (i.e., tumor mass). Likewise, the choice of therapy will depend on the stage of the disease (see Chapters 34, 35). The key problem is determining whether the disease is confined solely above the diaphragm (i.e., whether a *staging laparotomy* should be performed). The *principle of decision theory* teaches that additional testing should be undertaken only if management will differ upon obtaining the new information. Since management *does* differ between early and advanced states, and the noninvasive testing shown in Figure 33-1 can have false-negative or false-positive rates as high as 35%, deciding *when* to perform a staging laparotomy is important. The probabilistic approach to this decision in HD is shown in Figure 33-2. The staging laparotomy is rarely indicated in nonHodgkin's lymphoma, since chemotherapy is the initial treatment of choice even in the early stages of the disease.

Suggested Readings

Linden A, Zankovic R, Theissen P, Diehl V, Schicha H: Malignant lymphoma: bone marrow imaging versus biopsy. Radiology 173:335, 1989

Lister TA, Crowther D, Sutcliffe SB, et al.: Report of committee convened to discuss the evaluation and staging of patients with Hodgkin's disease: Costwolds meeting. J Clin Oncol 7:1630, 1989

Moormeier JA, Williams SF, Golomb HM: The staging of nonHodgkin's lymphomas. Semin Oncol 17:43, 1990

Raubitschek AF, Goffman T, Glatstein E: A staging of lymphomas: practical thoughts on impractical practices. J Natl Cancer Inst Monogr 10:13, 1990

Rutheford CJ, Desforges JF, Davies B, Barnett AI: The decision to perform staging laparotomy in symptomatic Hodgkin's disease. Br J Haematol 44:347, 1980

Schicha H, Franke M, Smolorz J, Linden A, Waters W, Diehl V: Diagnostic strategies and staging procedures for Hodgkin's lymphoma: bone marrow scintigraphy and magnetic resonance imaging. Recent Results Cancer Res 17:112, 1989

Urba WD, Longo DL: Hodgkin's disease. N Engl J Med 326:648, 1992

Zagonel V, Tirrell U, Vaccher E, et al.: Clinical and laboratory findings at presentation in persistent generalized lymphadenopathy *vs* malignant lymphoma. Cancer Detect Prev 12:225, 1988

34 Hodgkin's Disease: Treatment*

The treatment goal in *Hodgkin's disease* (HD) is a cure with minimum morbidity and long-range toxicity. Therefore, the principle of the risk/benefit estimate dominates clinical reasoning in the management of patients with HD. These estimates may be derived from the *inverse relationship between tumor burden and curability and between staging and the extent of treatment*. An optimal management, therefore, would include minimizing both the extent of treatment and the extent of staging. Figures 33-1 and 33-2 show an optimal approach to staging in Hodgkin's disease. The exact definition of stage of disease then forms a basis for the choice of treatment(s). Overall, the choice will depend on whether the patient is in an *early* stage (stage IA–IIB), *intermediate* stage (IIIA$_1$–IIIA$_2$B), or *advanced* stage (IVA–IVB).† An additional, separate category will comprise patients with *bulky disease*, such as a large mediastinal lymphadenopathy. The major treatment decision problem is when to use *radiation therapy* (XRT) and when to use *chemotherapy* (CRx) or a combined (XRT+CRx) modality approach. The second decision problem is the selection of a specific chemotherapy regimen from among the more than forty regimens described in the literature. Two other decision problems represent a choice of salvage treatment and management of a residual mass after completion of initial treatment.

Figure 34-1 shows a suggested approach to the choice of treatment type, tailored to a specific stage of the disease. The algorithm is constructed based upon the results of control trials described in the literature, tailoring the risk of treatment without compromising the curative potential of the selected therapy. Tables 34-1–34-3 show details of MOPP and ABVD regimens, which are the basis for all other chemotherapy regimens described in the literature. Figure 34-2 shows a decision analytic approach to the management of a residual mass after completion of initial treatment.

With contemporary management, 70–80% of patients may expect to be cured. An additional 15–20% who fail initial therapy will achieve a durable, complete response to secondary treatment, and the rest will succumb either to the disease or to the effects of continuous therapy.

---

*See chapter on diagnostic workup of lymphoma for further clinical and epidemiological information.

† The majority of authors consider the presence of B symptoms beyond stage II of very important significance; accordingly, advanced stages comprise all stages from IIB–IVB; we also accept this approach to HD, but singling out stage IIIA$_1$ as a separate category (see Fig. 34-1).

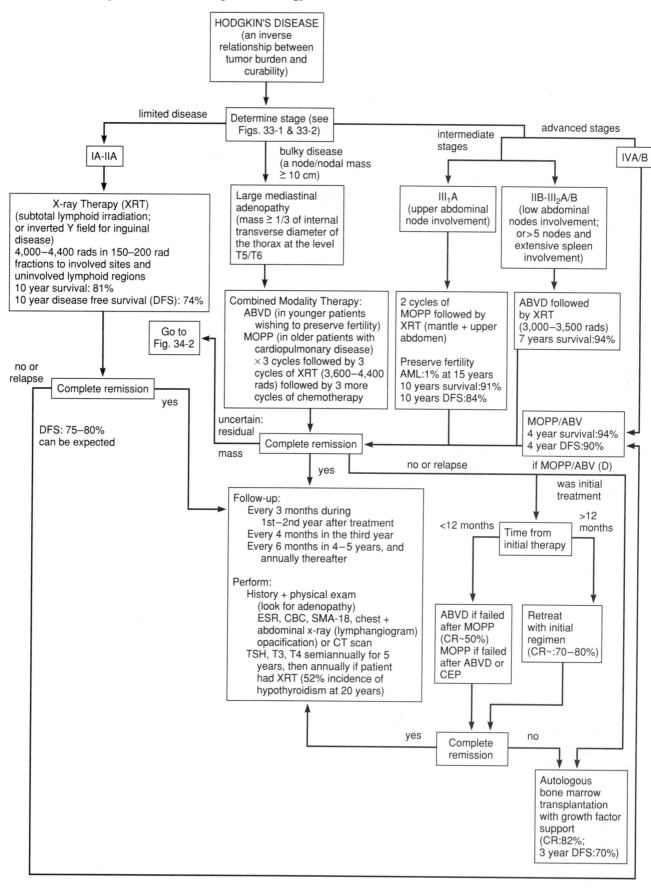

Table 34-1. MOPP and ABVD Regimens[a]

MOPP[b] (mg/m²)[c]	ABVD (mg/m²)[c]	MOPP/ABV (mg/m²)[d]
Mechlorethamine 6 IV on days 1, 8	*Doxorubicin* 25 IV on days 1, 15	*Mechlorethamine* 6 IV on day 1
Vincristine 1.4 IV on days 1, 8	*Bleomycin* 10 IV on days 1, 15	*Vincristine* 1.4 IV on day 1 (maximum 2.0 mg)
Procarbazine 100 PO on days 1–14	*Vinblastine* 6 IV on days 1, 15	*Procarbazine* 100 PO on days 1–7
Prednisone 40 mg PO on days 1–14	*Dacarbazine* 375 IV on days 1, 15	*Prednisone* 40 mg PO on days 1–14 *Doxorubicin* 35 IV on day 8 *Bleomycin* 10 IV on day 8 *Vinblastine* 6 iV on day 8

[a] Administer as many cycles as required to achieve full documented remission (this includes repetition of biopsies of tissues initially involved) followed by two additional cycles as treatment consolidation (usually 6 + 2 cycles); if patient progresses or does not respond at all after 2–3 cycles, consider it as a refractory disease; see Table 34-2 for sliding scale for drug dose adjustment based upon hematologic toxicities.
[b] MVPP: vinblastine (6 mg/m²) is substituted for vincristine. LOPP: chlorambucil (6 mg/m²) is substituted for mechlorethamine and vinblastine (6 mg/m²) for vincristine.
[c] Every 28 days
[d] Repeat every 28 days; see [a] for duration of therapy.

Table 34-2. Sliding Scale For Dose Adjustment of MOPP and ABVD Based Upon Hematologic Toxicity[a]

Leukocyte Count (/mm³)	Platelet Count (/mm³)	Dose Adjustment
>4,000	>100,000	100% all drugs
3,000–3,900	>100,000	100% vincristine,[b] 100% bleomycin; 75% mechlorethamine, 75% procarbazine (after MOPP only; 50% after hybrid program); 50% doxorubicin
2,000–2,900	50,000–100,000	100% vincristine; 25% mechlorethamine, 25% procarbazine 50% bleomycin; 25% doxorubicin
1,000–1,900	50,000–100,000	50% vincristine, 25% mechlorethamine, 25% procarbazine, 25% bleomycin, 25% doxorubicin
<1,000	<50,000	No drug

[a] Recent data indicates that G(M)-CSF in doses of 8 or 16 µg/kg for 5 days, administered on day 17 of the chemotherapy cycle improves hematologic recovery after MOPP, resulting in an increase in the overall tolerated dose of myelosuppressive drugs (see Housaard DJ and Nissen NI: J Clin Oncol 10:390, 1992) (for dose modification in case of hepatic dysfunction, see Table 22-3).
[b] If signs of peripheral neuropathy develop (inability to button clothes), dose is reduced to 50%; if patient develops ileus or has difficulty ambulating, vincristine should be held until symptoms improve, then resume at a 50% dose.

Fig. 34-1. Management of Hodgkin's disease (HD). The principle of the *risk/benefit estimate* dominates clinical reasoning in the management of patients with HD. The algorithm is constructed based upon the results of control trials described in the literature, tailoring risk of treatment without compromising the curative potential of the selected therapy. It should be noted that some investigators would use radiation therapy (XRT) in all early stages, and that others will use chemotherapy (CrX) in all stages. *Note*: Patients themselves will play an increasing role in decision management, since the treatment risk/benefit ratio could be highly individualized (e.g., wish for fertility or hair preservation, choice between alkylating agents and doxorubicin-containing regimens in patients over 50, etc.) See Tables 34-1–34-3 for details of MOPP and ABVD regimen, which are the basis for all other chemotherapy regimens described in the literature. (DFS, disease-free survival)

Table 34-3. Acute and Long-range Toxicities Associated With Current Treatment Modalities for Hodgkin's Disease

Short-term Toxicities	Long-term Toxicities
Mortality (~2–3%)	Male sterility (MOPP—90–100%, with 10–20% of recovery)
Vomiting[a] (almost 100%)	Amenorrhoea and premature ovarian failure (MOPP—75–85% in women >30 yrs; 20% in women <30 yrs)
Leukopenia (20–25%—MOPP; 40%—ABVD)	Pericarditis (XRT—15–30%)
Thrombocytopenia (15–20%—MOPP; 25%—ABVD)	Pneumonitis + chronic restrictive fibrosis (XRT—~20%)
Peripheral neuropathy (more with vincristine than with vinblastine)	Cardiomyopathy (doxorubicin—when dose >400–450 mg/m^2)
	Lung fibrosis (bleomycin—when dose >150 mg/m^2)
Alopecia (doxorubicin—56%; 30%—MOPP)	Acute leukemia (1–4% at 10 yr after MOPP 0.7% at 10 yr after ABVD 10–15% at 10 yr after XRT + MOPP)
Skin hyperpigmentation (19%—bleomycin)	NonHodgkin's lymphoma (2–4% at 10 yrs after chemotherapy)
	Solid tumors (13% at 15 years after XRT; continues to rise)

[a] Give antiemetics: e.g., metoclopramide 0.5 mg/kg IV over 10–15 min 30 min before chemotherapy + dexamethasone 10 mg IV (push) + diphenhydramine 50 mg IV (optional); repeat metoclopramide 0.5 mg/kg PO 2 hrs, 5 h, 8 hrs; dexamethasone PO 8 mg at 6 hrs, 12 hrs, 18 hrs. Or ondansetron IV 0.15 mg/kg in 50 ml of normal saline over 15 min beginning 30 min before chemotherapy; repeat at 4 and 8 hours after first dose.

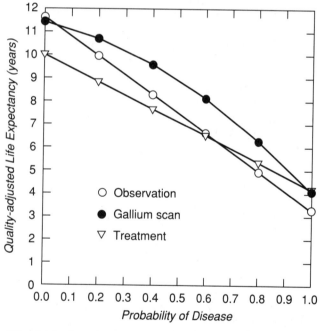

Fig. 34-2. Decision analysis of the management of a residual (mediastinal) mass after completion of initial treatment. At lower probabilities, observation is the preferred management; at a probability >3%, gallium scan is the best option. (From Djulbegovic et al.: Medical Hypotheses, Churchill Livingstone, Inc, 1992, with permission.)

Suggested Readings

Bonadonna G, Santoro A: Current issues in the management of advanced Hodgkin's disease. Blood Reviews 4:69, 1990

Canellos GP: Can MOPP be replaced in the treatment of advanced Hodgkin's disease? Semin Oncol 17:2, 1990

Guinee VF, Giacco GG, Durand M, et al.: The prognosis of Hodgkin's disease in older adults. J Clin Oncol 9:947, 1991

Henkelmann GC, Hagemeister FB, Fuller LM: Two cycles of MOPP and radiotherapy for stage III$_1$A and stage III$_1$B Hodgkin's disease. J Clin Oncol 6:1293, 1988

Hoppe RT: Early-stage Hodgkin's disease: a choice of treatments or a treatment of choice? J Clin Oncol 9:897, 1991

Hoppe RT: Development of effective salvage treatment programs for Hodgkin's disease: an ongoing clinical challenge. Blood 77:2093, 1991

Longo DL, Glatstein E, Duffey PL, et al.: Radiation therapy versus combination therapy in the treatment of early-stage Hodgkin's disease: seven-year results of a prospective randomized trial. J Clin Oncol 9:906, 1991

35 | NonHodgkin's Lymphomas: Treatment

The reasoning strategy upon which effective treatment decisions for *nonHodgkin's lymphoma* (NHL) are made is still based upon determination of *histological subtype* (see box in Chapter 33, p. 151) and *tumor burden* (i.e., stage of disease, see Tables 33-1 and 33-2). None of the other clinical, pathologic, immunologic, and (molecular) biologic information correlates better with the natural history of the disease and response to treatment.* Therefore, clinically speaking, NHL can be divided into three groups: (1) *low-grade lymphoma*, (2) *aggressive lymphomas*, and (3) *rapidly progressive high-grade lymphoma* (Fig. 35-1A). Management will further depend on whether the patient is in an *early* (Ia–IIa, absence of bulky disease and B symptoms) or an *advanced* stage (IIb–IVb, bulky disease) of disease.† Finally, the *anatomic site* of presentation, besides peripheral

---

*An impressive amount of information on the significance of T and B subtyping, various chromosome aberrations, the presence of specific oncogenes, and numerous other prognostic variables have not as yet translated into revised clinical management.

† Numerous ways of attempting to measure tumor mass have been described; final stage is usually produced upon the measurement of the number of sites involved, mass size, performance status, LDH level, and systemic symptoms. Overall, the Ann Arbor staging system is still more widely utilized than other systems and, therefore, is used in this chapter.

‡ These so-called special sites NHL (see Fig. 35-1E) are, by and large, characteristics of aggressive and rapidly progressive high-grade lymphomas; low-grade lymphomas, for example, do not involve testes or the central nervous system (CNS).

adenopathy, may play a key role in the choice of management (see Fig. 35-1E).‡

These pathophysiological principles are then coupled with an estimate of the probabilities of response, cure, and risk of specific types of treatment. Low-grade lymphomas, although indolent in their course, cannot be cured. There is no proof that *any* treatment changes the natural history of the disease, which is characterized by an overall 6–8 years median survival. The goal, therefore, is palliation and control of symptoms, with minimal induced treatment-related toxicity. Aggressive and high-grade lymphomas can, on the other hand, be cured, despite a rapid clinical course if left untreated (overall median survival: 1–3 years). The major decision dilemma in the treatment of aggressive NHL is the choice of an adequate chemotherapeutic regimen from among the more than twenty combinations currently in use. Randomized trials are currently in progress to provide an answer to this question, but decision analysis indicates that the best regimen is one that induces the highest remission rate and causes minimal late sequelae (Fig. 35-2). Figures 35-1A–F show an algorithm for management of NHL and the box below shows details of first-generation regimen CHOP, second-generation regimen MACE-MOPP, and third-generation regimens MACOP-B. Table 35-1 shows the operating characteristics of various diagnostic tests in detecting a relapse from aggressive types of NHL.

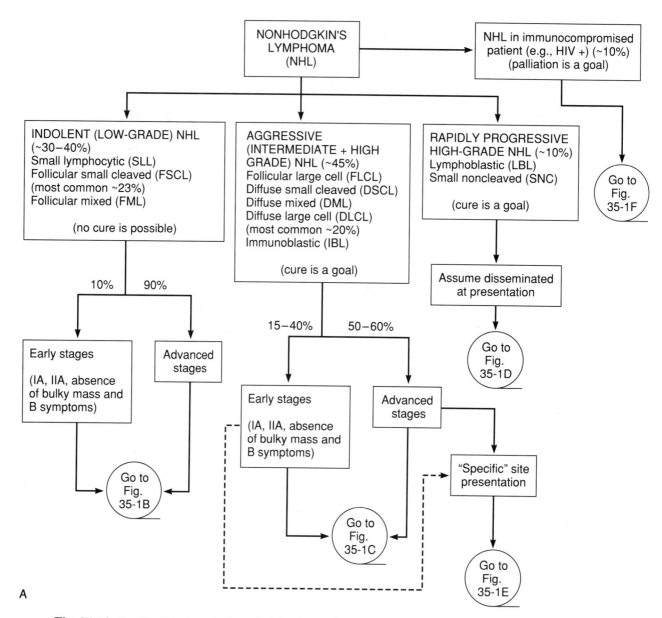

Fig. 35-1A–35-1F. Treatment of nonHodgkin's lymphomas (NHL). Reasoning principles are based upon understanding the *natural history of disease* (low grade *vs* aggressive *vs* rapidly progressive NHL), estimate of *tumor burden* upon presentation (stage of disease), and *probabilities of response, cure, and risk* of specific types of treatment. Presented is current literature consensus regarding treatment approach to NHL. *Abbreviations*: ABMT, autologous bone marrow transplantation; BM, bone marrow; DFS, disease-free survival; MS, median survival.

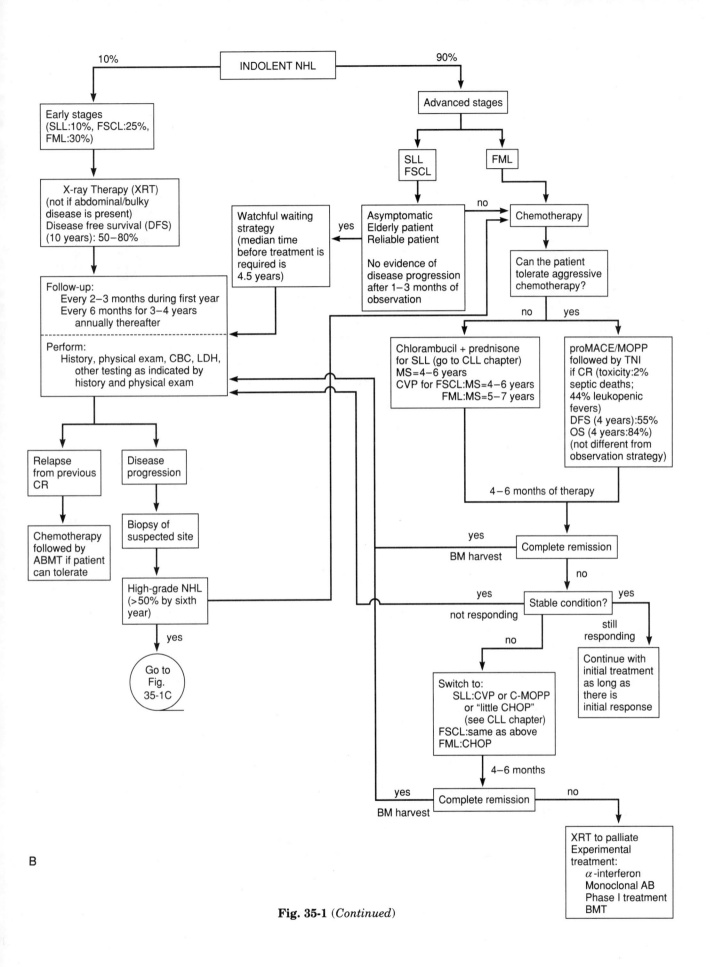

Fig. 35-1 (*Continued*)

B

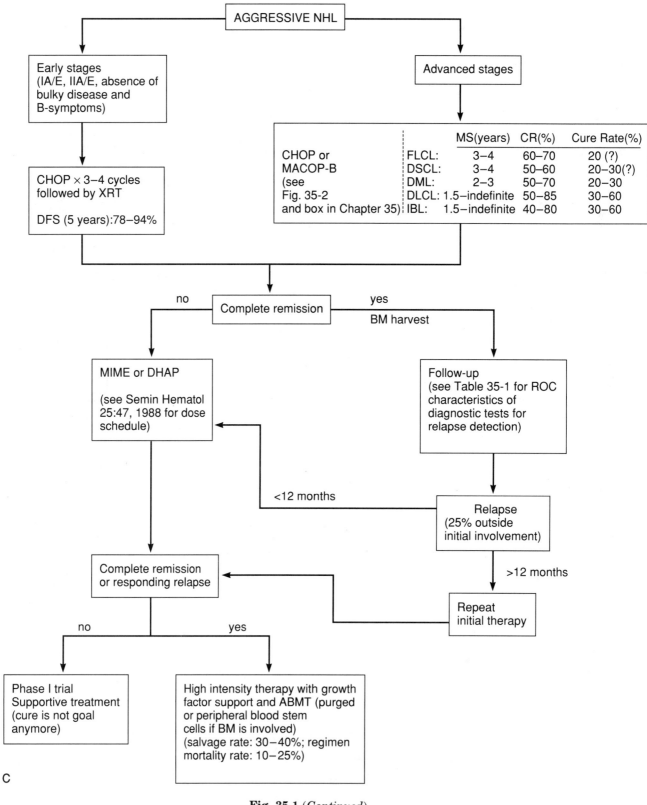

Fig. 35-1 (Continued)

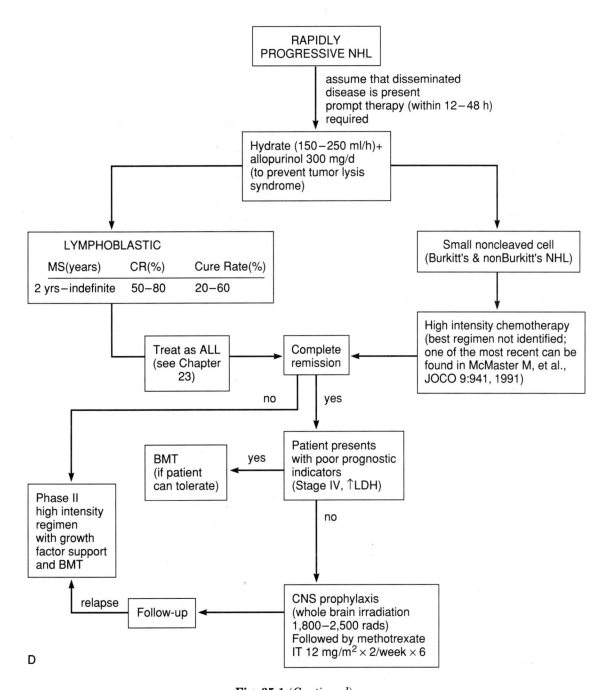

Fig. 35-1 (*Continued*)

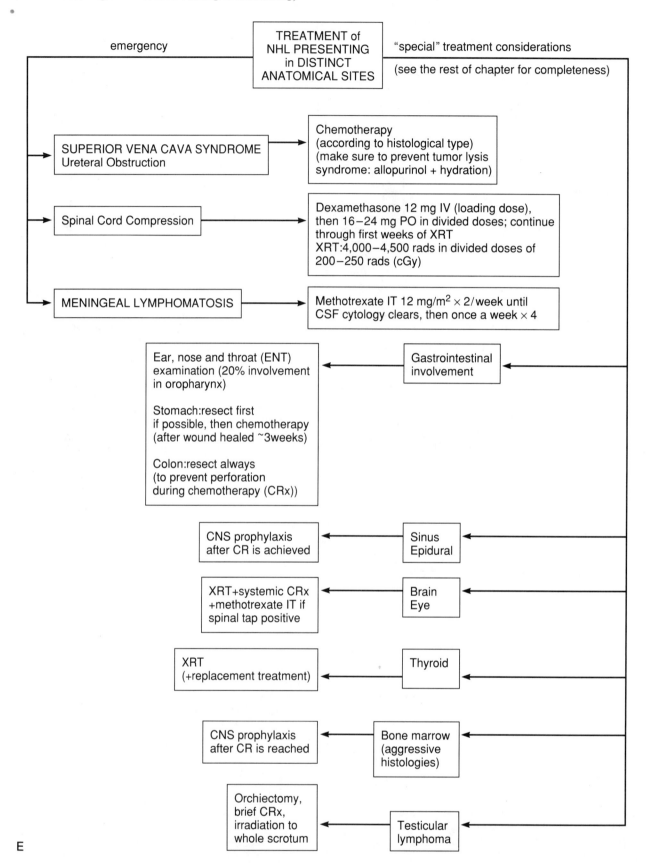

Fig. 35-1 (*Continued*)

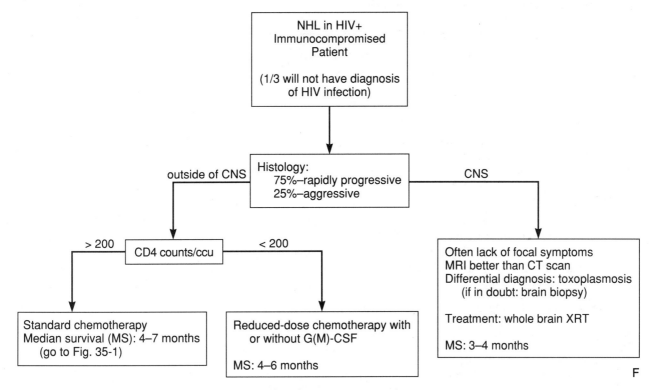

Fig. 35-1 (Continued)

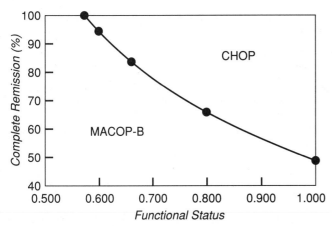

Fig. 35-2. Decision analysis of the treatment choice between the first generation regimen (CHOP) and the third generation regimen (MACOP-B). The choice of a particular regimen will depend on a combination of its complete remission (CR) rate and its effect upon functional status. New data seems to indicate that both regimens produce the same CR rate (~55%); an estimate of the regimen's effect on functional status then becomes a critical element in the choice between two regimens. (From Djulbegovic et al. Med Decis Making 11:1, 1991, with permission.) To use a nomogram, determine CR and functional status for a particular regimen. The choice of chemotherapy will depend on whether these two lines cross each other below or above "the line of indifference" (e.g., if CR for CHOP is 65% and functional status associated with it is 90%, then CHOP would become preferred regimen).

Table 35-1. Operating Characteristics of Diagnostic Tests in Detection of Relapse in Aggressive NonHodgkin's Lymphoma[a]

Diagnostic Test	Sensitivity (%)[b]	Specificity (%)
Physical exam	80	99
CBC count	21	98
LDH	65	85
Chest x-ray	21	95
Chest CT scan	45	83
Abdominal/pelvic CT/US	55	94
Gallium scan	90	90
Bone marrow aspirate/biopsy	26	100

[a] Data from Weeks et al.: JOCO 9:1196, 1991, with permission. Probability of relapse (after M/m BACOD therapy) is 2.1% per year for early stages; in advanced stages this increases to 13.3%/year for the first 2 years, 7.7% per year for years 2–5, and 1.6% per year of relapse thereafter; these probabilities may be used as pretest estimates, which can be combined with the values below to obtain post-test probability of relapse (see also Chapter 1).

[b] At the time of relapse; sensitivity as a screening test (performed within 3 months before clinical relapse) is notoriously low, ranging from 0 for chest CT to 42% for elevated LDH.

First-Generation Chemotherapy Regimen: CHOP[a]

Cyclophosphamide	750 mg/m^2 IV on day 1[b]
Doxorubicin	50 mg/m^2 IV on day 1
Vincristine	1.4 mg/m^2 on day 1
Prednisone	100 mg PO on days 1–5

Second-Generation Regimen: proMACE-MOPP

Prednisone 6 mg/m^2 PO days 1–14
Methotrexate 1,500 mg/m^2 IV on day 15 (followed by leucovorin rescue 24 h after MTX)
Adriamycin 25 mg/m^2 IV on days 1, 8 IV
Cyclophosphamide 650 mg/m^2 IV on days 1, 8
Etoposide 120 mg/m^2 IV on days 1, 8
(Repeat this schedule q 28 days and then give MOPP—Table 34.1—after maximal response is achieved)
(see Fisher et al: Ann Intern Med 98:304, 1983 for details)

Third-Generation Regimen: MACOP-B[c]

Methotrexate (MTX) 400 mg/m^2 IV on weeks 2, 6, 10 (100 mg as a bolus, remaining 300 infused over 4 h)
Folinic acid 15 mg PO q 6 h × 6 (24 h from MTX)
Doxorubicin 50 mg/m^2 IV on weeks 1, 3, 5, 7, 9, 11
Cyclophosphamide 350 mg/m^2 IV on wk 1, 3, 5, 7, 9, 11
Vincristine 1.4 mg/m^2 IV on wk 2, 4, 6, 8, 10, 12 (maximum 2 mg)
Bleomycin 10 U/m^2 IV on wk 4, 8, 12 (hydrocortisone 100 mg IV just before bleomycin)
Prednisone 75 mg PO q d, dose tapered over the last 14 days
Cotrimoxazole (Trimethoprim sulfamethoxazole) 2 DS tbl PO daily throughout
Ketoconazole 200 mg PO daily throughout
Cytarabine 30 mg/m^2 IT twice a week × 6 (CNS prophylaxis after CR is achieved in patients with aggressive lymphoma involving bone marrow or sinus)

---

[a] Repeat every 21–28 days depending upon CBC; administer as many cycles as required to achieve full, documented remission (this includes repetition of biopsies of tissues initially involved)), followed by 2 additional cycles as treatment consolidation (usually 6 + 2 cycles); if patient progresses or does not respond at all after 2–3 cycles, consider it as a refractory disease; rapidly responding patients have more durable remissions. (Data from Armitage et al.: J Clin Oncol 2:898, 1984.)

[b] Reduce dose to 50% if white blood cells (WBC) 3,000–4,000/mm^3 or to 25% if WBC is 2,000–3,000 and/or platelets 50,000–100,000/mm^3; do not give therapy for lower values of WBC or platelets; see Table 34-2 for the comment on the use of growth factors in this setting; note that G(M)-CSF may be used to boost up counts.

[c] Dose modification: full dose if absolute granulocyte counts >1,000/mm^3; reduce dose of cyclophosphamide and doxorubicin (not other drugs) to 65% of dose if granulocyte counts are 100–999; delay therapy for a week if counts <100, administer platelet transfusion to keep platelets >10,000/mm^3 (no dose modification necessary) (Data from Klimo and Connors: Semin Hematol 24:26, 1987.)

Suggested Readings

Armitage JO: Bone marrow transplantation in the treatment of patients with lymphoma. Blood 73:1749, 1989

DeVita VT, Hubbard SM, Young RC, Longo DL: The role of chemotherapy in diffuse aggressive lymphoma. Semin Hematol 25:2, 1988

Djulbegovic B, Hollenberg J, Woodcock TM, Herzig R: Comparison of different treatment strategies for diffuse large-cell lymphomas. Med Decis Making 11:1, 1991

Kwark LW, Wilson M, Weiss LM, et al.: Similar outcome of treatment of B cell and T cell diffuse large-cell lymphomas: The Stanford experience. J Clin Oncol 9:1426, 1991

Longo DL: Combined modality therapy for localized aggressive lymphoma: enough or too much? J Clin Oncol 7:1179, 1989

Weeks JC, Yeap BY, Canellos GP, Shipp MA: Value of follow-up procedures in patients with large-cell lymphoma who achieve a complete remission. J Clin Oncol 9:1196, 1991

Yl PI, Coleman M, Saltz L, et al.: Chemotherapy of large cell lymphoma: status update. Semin Oncol 17:60, 1990

Young RC, Longo DL, Glastein E, Ihde DC, Jaffe ES, DeVita VT: The treatment of indolent lymphomas: watchful waiting versus aggressive combined modality treatment. Semin Hematol 25:11, 1988

36 Cutaneous T Cell Lymphoma

The spectrum of *cutaneous T cell lymphoma* includes three similar but distinct entities: (1) *mycosis fungoides* (MF), (2) *Sézary* syndrome (SS), an erythrodermic variant associated with a leukemic phase of the disease (typical cerebriform cells of SS are usually found in the buffy coat), and (3) *human T cell leukemia/lymphoma*, a rare disease associated with bone lesions, hypercalcemia, and HTLV-I virus infection. MF and SS are the most common primary lymphomas of the skin with an incidence that is increasing from 0.2 cases per 100,000 population in 1974 to 0.4 cases per 100,000 population in 1984. The diagnosis of MF/SS is based upon the histopathology of the skin, characterized by dermal infiltrates of atypical lymphocytes with pathognomonic Pautrier's microabscesses. The majority of cases of MF/SS are of the T helper phenotype (CD4 +).

MF and SS are disorders with a chronic course, and survival strongly correlates with tumor burden. Staging is, therefore, essential in the clinical management of these patients. Figure 36-1 shows a staging system, recommended staging procedures, and survival according to the stage of disease. It is thought that MF initially involves the skin and, with time, disseminates to lymph nodes, the spleen, the liver, or other visceral organs. In general, patients who comprise a good-risk group are those with skin plaque-lesions only and who have a median survival over 12 years. The intermediate-risk group

have disease that *has* spread to nodes or blood but *without* visceral involvement or node effacement; they have a median survival of about 5 years. The poor-risk group of patients have visceral involvement or node effacement, and their median survival is about 2.5 years. Infection, usually from the skin (*Staphylococcus aureus* and *Pseudomonas aeruginosa*), is the major cause of death (50%).

Disseminated disease is found in about 50% of patients at initial presentation if staging is done by routine labs and imaging studies. A bone marrow aspirate/biopsy is positive in about 20% of cases and is usually done only in patients with advanced stages; an abdominal CT is not helpful in early stages of these diseases. If, however, molecular biology techniques are employed in looking for clonal T cell gene rearrangement, then disseminated disease can be detected in more than 90% of patients. This forms a rationale for early aggressive treatment of cutaneous T cell lymphomas. Unfortunately, trials comparing aggressive chemotherapy as an initial treatment with conservative treatment did not improve the prognosis of these patients. Therefore, until new modalities are developed, one should probably favor topical treatment for localized disease and systemic chemotherapy for disseminated disease. This was the main rationale in the construction of the algorithm presented in Figure 36-2.

169

Staging Systems for Mycosis Fungoides

T stage
T1: Limited plaque, less than 10% body surface area
T2: Generalized plaque, 10% or greater of body
    surface area
T3: Cutaneous tumor (one or more)
T4: Erythroderma (generalized)

Adenopathy
Ad +: Palpable adenopathy
Ad −: No palpable adenopathy

Lymph node class (biopsy)
LN1: Reactive node
LN2: Dermatopathic node, small clusters of
    convoluted cells
LN3: Dermatopathic node, large clusters of
    convoluted cells
LN4: Lymph node effacement

Visceral
V+: Positive visceral biopsy
V−: Negative visceral biopsy

Stages*
IA: T1; Ad−; LN1, LN2, V−
IB: T2; Ad−; LN1, LN2, V−
IIA: T1, T2; Ad + ; LN1, LN2; V−
IIB: T3; Ad ±; LN1, LN2; V−
III: T4; Ad ±; LN1, LN2, V−
IVA: T1-T4; Ad ±; LN3 or LN4; V−
IVB: T1-T4; Ad±; LN1-LN4; V+

Blood
B+: Positive blood smear
B−: Negative blood smear

Modified Staging Evaluation of Mycosis Fungoides and the Sézary Syndrome*

Positive skin biopsy
Skin examination for T class
Node examination
    Adenopathy
    Biopsy
Peripheral blood smear and cell size
Visceral biopsy (marrow, liver if node examination or
    peripheral blood smear was positive)
Prognostic groups
    Low risk
        T1 or T2; LN1, LN2; negative peripheral blood
        smear; negative visceral biopsy
    Intermediate risk
        Not encompassed by low or high
    High risk
        LN4 or positive visceral biopsy

*T1-T4 = T stages of skin disease (38); LN1-LN4 = grade 1 to 4 lymph node histopathologic findings (35).

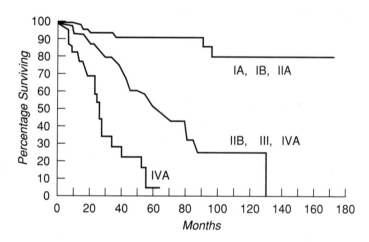

Fig. 36-1. Staging system, recommended procedures, and survival according to stage of disease in mycosis fungoides/Sézary syndrome. (From Sausville, Eddy, Makuch, et al.: Ann Intern Med 109:372, 1989, with permission.)

Fig. 36-2. An algorithm for the treatment of mycosis fungoides/Sézary syndrome. Rationale for the recommended strategy is based upon information that initial aggressive chemotherapy does not improve the prognosis of these patients, but causes greater toxicity. Therefore, according to the *risk/benefit* principles, the sequence of palliative therapies remains the treatment of choice in this long-lasting but deadly disease. *Abbreviations*: COP—Cyclophosphamide, Oncovin (Vincristin), prednisone; CHOP—cyclophosphamide, doxorubicin, Oncovin (Vincristin), prednisone; HTLV-1—human T cell lymphoma virus; ABMT—autologous bone marrow transplantation.

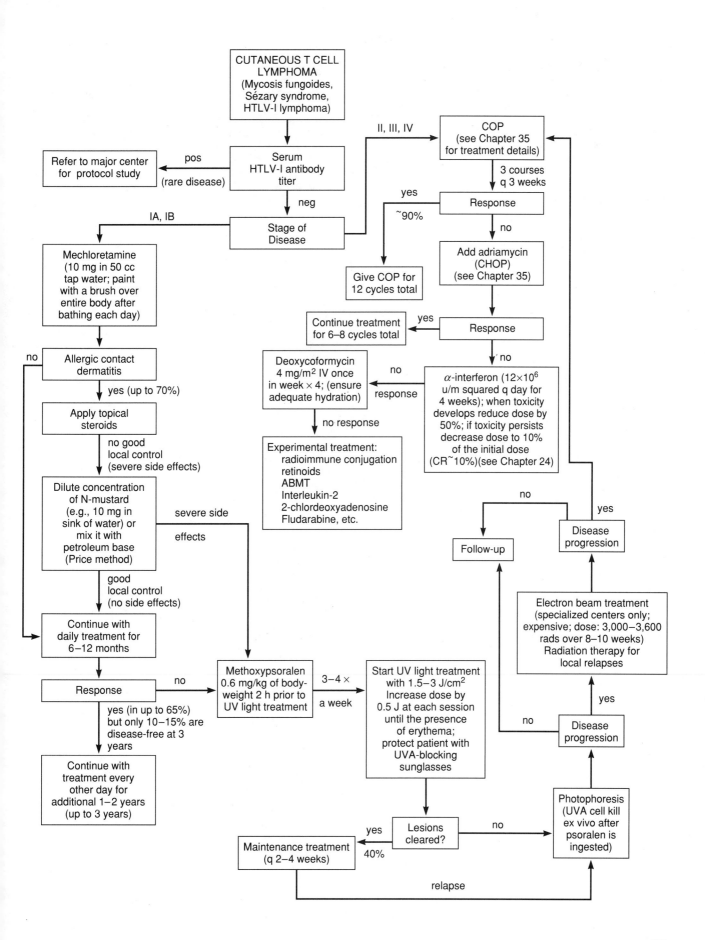

CUTANEOUS T CELL LYMPHOMA
(Mycosis fungoides,
Sézary syndrome,
HTLV-I lymphoma)

Serum HTLV-I antibody titer

pos → Refer to major center for protocol study
(rare disease)

neg

Stage of Disease

IA, IB

II, III, IV → COP (see Chapter 35 for treatment details)

3 courses q 3 weeks

Response

yes ~90% → Give COP for 12 cycles total

no → Add adriamycin (CHOP) (see Chapter 35)

Response

yes → Continue treatment for 6–8 cycles total

no → α-interferon (12×10⁶ u/m squared q day for 4 weeks); when toxicity develops reduce dose by 50%; if toxicity persists decrease dose to 10% of the initial dose (CR~10%)(see Chapter 24)

Deoxycoformycin 4 mg/m² IV once in week × 4; (ensure adequate hydration)

no response → Experimental treatment: radioimmune conjugation, retinoids, ABMT, Interleukin-2, 2-chlordeoxyadenosine, Fludarabine, etc.

Mechloretamine (10 mg in 50 cc tap water; paint with a brush over entire body after bathing each day)

Allergic contact dermatitis

no →

yes (up to 70%)

Apply topical steroids

no good local control (severe side effects)

Dilute concentration of N-mustard (e.g., 10 mg in sink of water) or mix it with petroleum base (Price method)

severe side effects →

good local control (no side effects)

Continue with daily treatment for 6–12 months

Response

no → Methoxypsoralen 0.6 mg/kg of bodyweight 2 h prior to UV light treatment

3–4 × a week → Start UV light treatment with 1.5–3 J/cm² Increase dose by 0.5 J at each session until the presence of erythema; protect patient with UVA-blocking sunglasses

yes (in up to 65%) but only 10–15% are disease-free at 3 years

Continue with treatment every other day for additional 1–2 years (up to 3 years)

Lesions cleared?

yes 40% → Maintenance treatment (q 2–4 weeks)

no → Photophoresis (UVA cell kill ex vivo after psoralen is ingested)

relapse →

Disease progression

no → Follow-up

yes → Electron beam treatment (specialized centers only; expensive; dose: 3,000–3,600 rads over 8–10 weeks) Radiation therapy for local relapses

Disease progression

no → Follow-up

yes → Disease progression

no →

yes →

Suggested Readings

Hallahan DE, Griem ML, Griem SF, et al.: Combined modality therapy for tumor stage mycosis fungoides: results of a 10-year follow-up. J Clin Oncol 6:1177, 1988

Kaye FJ, Bunn PA, Steinberg SM, et al.: A randomized trial comparing combination electron-beam radiation and chemotherapy with topical therapy in the initial treatment of mycosis fungoides. N Engl J Med 321:1784, 1989

Kuzel TM, Roenigk HH, Rosen ST: Mycosis fungoides and the Sézary syndrome: a review of pathogenesis, diagnosis, and therapy. J Clin Oncol 9:1298, 1991

Sausville EA, Eddy JL, Makuch RW, et al.: Histopathologic staging at initial diagnosis of mycosis fungoides and the Sézary syndrome. Definitions of three distinctive prognostic groups. Ann Intern Med 109:372, 1989

Young RC: Mycosis fungoides. The therapeutic search continues. N Engl J Med 321:1822, 1989

37 Plasma Cell Disorders

Plasma cell disorders, or monoclonal gammopathies, are clinically and biochemically diverse disorders that share two major features: first, an uncontrolled proliferation of the lymphocyte-plasma cell series, and second, the production of a large amount of electrophoretically and immunologically homogeneous immunoglobulin. Monoclonal protein (M-protein) is usually detected as a sharp peak or spike in the beta or gamma globulin zone on serum electrophoresis. Electrophoresis on a cellulose acetate membrane is useful for screening purposes, although agarose is more sensitive in detecting small monoclonal bands. After screening, immunoelectrophoretic and/or immunofixation should be used to confirm the presence of monoclonal protein, and to determine its heavy and light chain type.

Monoclonal immunoglobulins ("monoclonal gammopathies") are seen in a variety of clinical states, the most common being: (1) monoclonal gammopathy of undetermined significance (MGUS)—67%, (2) multiple myeloma (MM)—13.5%, and (3) primary amyloidosis—9%. Less common associations are lymphoma and other lymphoproliferative diseases (5%), Waldenström's macroglobulinemia (2%), chronic lymphatic leukemia (2%), smoldering multiple myeloma (SMM) (0.9%), and solitary or extramedullary plasmacytoma 0.5%.

The most common types of M-protein produced by plasma cell neoplasms are IgG—52%, IgA—21%, and IgM—12%; in 11% of patients there is an excretion of light chain only, and IgD is found in 2%. Heavy chain diseases comprise less than 1%, and IgE < 0.01%.

The most important information needed for diagnosis in patients with monoclonal gammopathy are: (1) the percentage of plasma cells in a bone marrow aspirate/biopsy, (2) immunologic identification and measurement of serum/urine M-protein, and (3) radiology of the axial skeleton (skull, vertebral bodies, ribs, and pelvis).

This may lead to definition of the following *production rule*: *If* patient is older than 40 years of age *and* has **unexplained** anemia/renal insufficiency/bone pain, *then* suspect plasma cell disorders (go to Fig. 37-1). The above-mentioned relative frequencies will dictate the likelihood of a specific clinical diagnosis. Figure 37-1 shows an approach to diagnosis that is highly deterministic, based upon definition of important clinical features of the condition considered. It is also combined with a physiologic principle of considering a differential diagnosis along the line of an immunologic subtype of monoclonal protein (i.e., IgG *vs* IgM *vs* IgA *vs* IgD and IgE).

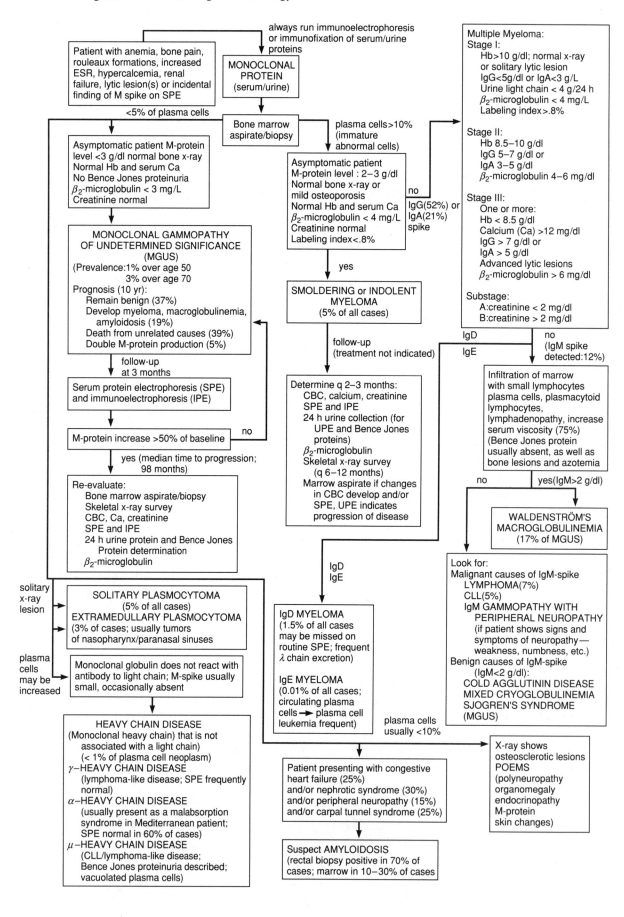

always run immunoelectrophoresis or immunofixation of serum/urine proteins

Patient with anemia, bone pain, rouleaux formations, increased ESR, hypercalcemia, renal failure, lytic lesion(s) or incidental finding of M spike on SPE

MONOCLONAL PROTEIN (serum/urine)

<5% of plasma cells

Bone marrow aspirate/biopsy

plasma cells >10% (immature abnormal cells)

Asymptomatic patient M-protein level <3 g/dl normal bone x-ray Normal Hb and serum Ca No Bence Jones proteinuria β_2-microglobulin < 3 mg/L Creatinine normal

Asymptomatic patient M-protein level : 2–3 g/dl Normal bone x-ray or mild osteoporosis Normal Hb and serum Ca β_2-microglobulin < 4 mg/L Creatinine normal Labeling index <.8%

Multiple Myeloma:
Stage I:
Hb >10 g/dl; normal x-ray or solitary lytic lesion IgG<5g/dl or IgA<3 g/L Urine light chain < 4 g/24 h β_2-microglobulin < 4 mg/L Labeling index >.8%

Stage II:
Hb 8.5–10 g/dl IgG 5–7 g/dl or IgA 3–5 g/L β_2-microglobulin 4–6 mg/dl

Stage III:
One or more: Hb < 8.5 g/dl Calcium (Ca) >12 mg/dl IgG > 7 g/dl or IgA > 5 g/dl Advanced lytic lesions β_2-microglobulin > 6 mg/dl

Substage:
A:creatinine < 2 mg/dl B:creatinine > 2 mg/dl

no
IgG(52%) or IgA(21%) spike

MONOCLONAL GAMMOPATHY OF UNDETERMINED SIGNIFICANCE (MGUS)
(Prevalence:1% over age 50
3% over age 70
Prognosis (10 yr):
Remain benign (37%)
Develop myeloma, macroglobulinemia, amyloidosis (19%)
Death from unrelated causes (39%)
Double M-protein production (5%)

yes

SMOLDERING or INDOLENT MYELOMA
(5% of all cases)

IgD
IgE

no
(IgM spike detected:12%)

follow-up at 3 months

follow-up (treatment not indicated)

Serum protein electrophoresis (SPE) and immunoelectrophoresis (IPE)

Infiltration of marrow with small lymphocytes plasma cells, plasmacytoid lymphocytes, lymphadenopathy, increase serum viscosity (75%) (Bence Jones protein usually absent, as well as bone lesions and azotemia

no

M-protein increase >50% of baseline

no

Determine q 2–3 months:
CBC, calcium, creatinine SPE and IPE
24 h urine collection (for UPE and Bence Jones proteins)
β_2-microglobulin
Skeletal x-ray survey (q 6–12 months)
Marrow aspirate if changes in CBC develop and/or SPE, UPE indicates progression of disease

yes (median time to progression; 98 months)

yes(IgM>2 g/dl)

Re-evaluate:
Bone marrow aspirate/biopsy
Skeletal x-ray survey
CBC, Ca, creatinine
SPE and IPE
24 h urine protein and Bence Jones Protein determination
β_2-microglobulin

WALDENSTRÖM'S MACROGLOBULINEMIA (17% of MGUS)

IgD
IgE

Look for:
Malignant causes of IgM-spike
LYMPHOMA(7%)
CLL(5%)
IgM GAMMOPATHY WITH PERIPHERAL NEUROPATHY
(if patient shows signs and symptoms of neuropathy—weakness, numbness, etc.)
Benign causes of IgM-spike
(IgM<2 g/dl):
COLD AGGLUTININ DISEASE
MIXED CRYOGLOBULINEMIA
SJOGREN'S SYNDROME
(MGUS)

solitary x-ray lesion

SOLITARY PLASMOCYTOMA (5% of all cases)
EXTRAMEDULLARY PLASMOCYTOMA (3% of cases; usually tumors of nasopharynx/paranasal sinuses

IgD MYELOMA
(1.5% of all cases may be missed on routine SPE; frequent λ chain excretion)

IgE MYELOMA
(0.01% of all cases; circulating plasma cells → plasma cell leukemia frequent)

plasma cells may be increased

Monoclonal globulin does not react with antibody to light chain; M-spike usually small, occasionally absent

plasma cells usually <10%

X-ray shows osteosclerotic lesions
POEMS
(polyneuropathy organomegaly endocrinopathy M-protein skin changes)

HEAVY CHAIN DISEASE
(Monoclonal heavy chain) that is not associated with a light chain)
(< 1% of plasma cell neoplasm)
γ–HEAVY CHAIN DISEASE
(lymphoma-like disease; SPE frequently normal)
α–HEAVY CHAIN DISEASE
(usually present as a malabsorption syndrome in Mediterranean patient; SPE normal in 60% of cases)
μ–HEAVY CHAIN DISEASE
(CLL/lymphoma-like disease; Bence Jones proteinuria described; vacuolated plasma cells)

Patient presenting with congestive heart failure (25%) and/or nephrotic syndrome (30%) and/or peripheral neuropathy (15%) and/or carpal tunnel syndrome (25%)

Suspect AMYLOIDOSIS
(rectal biopsy positive in 70% of cases; marrow in 10–30% of cases

Suggested Readings

Barlogie B, Epstein J, Selvanayagam P, Alexanian R: Plasma cell myeloma—new biological insight and advances in therapy. Blood 73:865, 1989

Greipp PR: Monoclonal gammopathies: new approaches to clinical problems in diagnosis and prognosis. Blood Rev 3:222, 1989

Knowling M, Harwood A, Bergsagel DE: A comparison of extramedullary plasmacytomas with multiple and solitary plasma cell tumors of bone. J Clin Oncol 1:255, 1983

Kyle RA, Lust JA: Monoclonal gammopathies of undetermined significance. Semin Hematol 26:176, 1989

Fig. 37-1. Diagnostic approach to monoclonal gammopathies. The workup starts with a *production rule*: a diagnosis of plasma cell disorders should be triggered in any patient over the age of 40 years with unexplained anemia, renal insufficiency, osteoporosis, an elevated sedimentation rate, radicular pain, discrete osteolytic bone lesions in the skeleton, polyneuropathy, or recurrent infections. The conditions are listed according to the probabilities of their diagnosis in the general population. The algorithm assumes that every patient will, as a minimum, have determination of: (1) the percentage of plasma cells in a bone marrow aspirate/biopsy, (b) immunologic identification and measurement of serum/urine M-protein, (c) skeletal x-ray survey. The diagnostic effectiveness is further increased if a *physiologic principle* of considering a differential diagnosis along the line of an immunologic subtype of monoclonal protein (i.e., IgG *vs* IgM *vs* IgA *vs* IgD and IgE) is applied as well. *Abbreviations*: SPE, serum protein electrophoresis; UPE, urine protein electrophoresis; IPE, immunoelectrophoresis; ESR, erythrocyte sedimentation rate.

38 | Multiple Myeloma

Multiple myeloma is a disease characterized by the neoplastic proliferation of a single clone of plasma cells. Its incidence is about 3–5 per 100,000 population; it is the most common hematologic malignancy in blacks, with an incidence of about 9.6 per 100,000. Overall, it comprises about 1% of all malignancies and about 10% of all hematologic malignancies. Multiple myeloma (MM) should be suspected in any patient older than 40 (only 2% younger than 40 suffer from myeloma) with unexplained anemia, renal dysfunction, or bone lesions (see Chapter 37). A clinical suspicion is confirmed by matching findings with diagnostic criteria (*deterministic principle*). The classic diagnostic triad is: >10% of immature plasma cells (the most specific test, virtually 100%) + M-protein in serum/urine + osteolytic lesions (see Fig. 37-1 for diagnostic workup). About 60% of patients will produce a monoclonal IgG protein, 20% IgA, 10% will be light chain excretors only (Bence Jones proteins), and the rest will be accounted for by IgD, IgE, and IgM monoclonal productions. Serum protein electrophoresis (SPE) will detect M-spike in about 75% of patients, but immunoelectrophoresis (IPE) of serum and urine proteins will detect 98–99% of cases (1–2% of cases are nonsecretors). In other words, negative IPE and UPE virtually excludes MM. Bone surveys will show lytic lesions in about 80% of cases (radionucleotide scan is inferior to x-ray and should not be ordered).

Tumor mass in myeloma correlates with clinical stages (see Fig. 37-1) in such a way that patients with stage III have more than 1 kg of tumor in the body (1.2×10^{12} cells/m^2), those with stage I have less than 0.5 kg of tumor ($<0.6 \times 10^{12}$ cells/m^2), and

patients with stage II have an amount of tumor in between these two extremes. The major clinical decisions in the treatment of myeloma are:

1. *Whether to treat.* Patients with *smoldering* or *indolent multiple myeloma* do not require treatment, and should not be treated unless progression occurs. This rationale is based upon the low probability of progression toward more advanced stages (2%/year). Symptomatic patients or patients with advanced stages should be treated.
2. *How to treat.* Patients with *solitary myeloma of the bone* (5% of all cases) should be treated with irradiation in the range of 4,000–5,000 rads. Lesions, however, remain solitary in about 15% of cases; therefore, careful follow-up is indicated (see below). *Extramedullary plasmocytoma* (3% of patients) can be controlled by irradiation and/or surgical resection. Patients with *symptomatic overt myeloma* should be treated with chemotherapy. Complex chemotherapy regimens have not proven to be more effective than standard treatment with melphalan-prednisone.
3. *How to follow treatment effects.* M-spike (as determined by IPE or SPE if M-spike is visible) highly correlates with tumor mass and is a primary test to follow. Recently, β_2-microglobulin is said to correlate with tumor mass even better, and

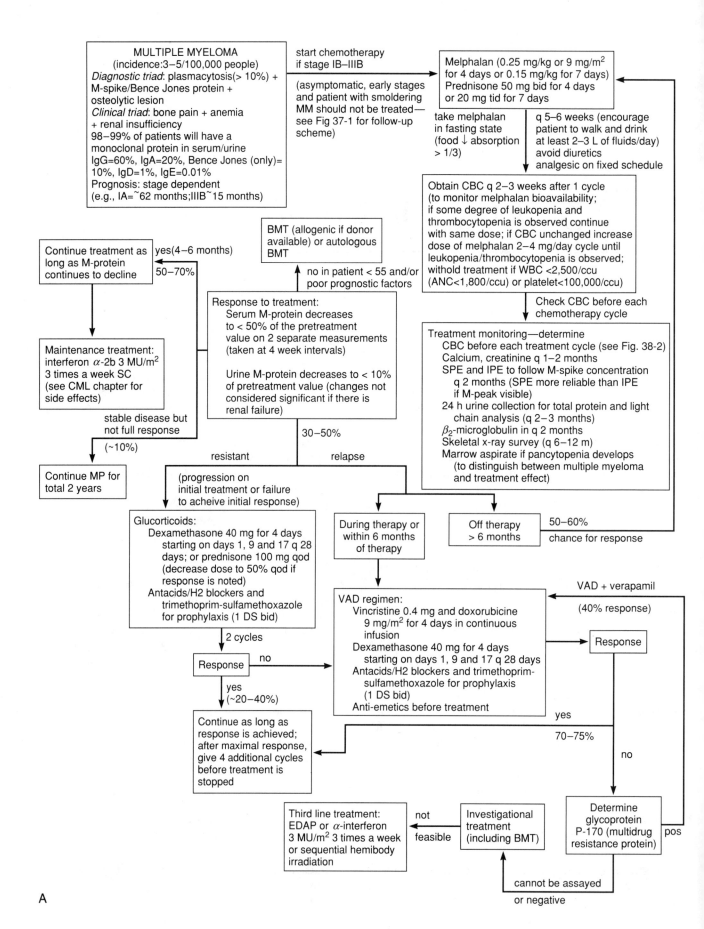

MULTIPLE MYELOMA
(incidence:3–5/100,000 people)
Diagnostic triad: plasmacytosis(> 10%) +
M-spike/Bence Jones protein +
osteolytic lesion
Clinical triad: bone pain + anemia
+ renal insufficiency
98–99% of patients will have a
monoclonal protein in serum/urine
IgG=60%, IgA=20%, Bence Jones (only)=
10%, IgD=1%, IgE=0.01%
Prognosis: stage dependent
(e.g., IA=~62 months;IIIB~15 months)

start chemotherapy
if stage IB–IIIB

(asymptomatic, early stages
and patient with smoldering
MM should not be treated—
see Fig 37-1 for follow-up
scheme)

Melphalan (0.25 mg/kg or 9 mg/m^2
for 4 days or 0.15 mg/kg for 7 days)
Prednisone 50 mg bid for 4 days
or 20 mg tid for 7 days

take melphalan
in fasting state
(food ↓ absorption
> 1/3)

q 5–6 weeks (encourage
patient to walk and drink
at least 2–3 L of fluids/day)
avoid diuretics
analgesic on fixed schedule

Obtain CBC q 2–3 weeks after 1 cycle
(to monitor melphalan bioavailability;
if some degree of leukopenia and
thrombocytopenia is observed continue
with same dose; if CBC unchanged increase
dose of melphalan 2–4 mg/day cycle until
leukopenia/thrombocytopenia is observed;
withold treatment if WBC <2,500/ccu
(ANC<1,800/ccu) or platelet<100,000/ccu)

Check CBC before each
chemotherapy cycle

Treatment monitoring—determine
CBC before each treatment cycle (see Fig. 38-2)
Calcium, creatinine q 1–2 months
SPE and IPE to follow M-spike concentration
q 2 months (SPE more reliable than IPE
if M-peak visible)
24 h urine collection for total protein and light
chain analysis (q 2–3 months)
β_2-microglobulin in q 2 months
Skeletal x-ray survey (q 6–12 m)
Marrow aspirate if pancytopenia develops
(to distinguish between multiple myeloma
and treatment effect)

Continue treatment as
long as M-protein
continues to decline

yes(4–6 months)
50–70%

BMT (allogenic if donor
available) or autologous
BMT

no in patient < 55 and/or
poor prognostic factors

Maintenance treatment:
interferon α-2b 3 MU/m^2
3 times a week SC
(see CML chapter for
side effects)

Response to treatment:
Serum M-protein decreases
to < 50% of the pretreatment
value on 2 separate measurements
(taken at 4 week intervals)

Urine M-protein decreases to < 10%
of pretreatment value (changes not
considered significant if there is
renal failure)

stable disease but
not full response
(~10%)

Continue MP for
total 2 years

resistant

(progression on
initial treatment or failure
to acheive initial response)

30–50%

relapse

During therapy or
within 6 months
of therapy

Off therapy
> 6 months

50–60%
chance for response

Glucorticoids:
Dexamethasone 40 mg for 4 days
starting on days 1, 9 and 17 q 28
days; or prednisone 100 mg qod
(decrease dose to 50% qod if
response is noted)
Antacids/H2 blockers and
trimethoprim-sulfamethoxazole
for prophylaxis (1 DS bid)

2 cycles

Response   no

yes
(~20–40%)

VAD regimen:
Vincristine 0.4 mg and doxorubicine
9 mg/m^2 for 4 days in continuous
infusion
Dexamethasone 40 mg for 4 days
starting on days 1, 9 and 17 q 28 days
Antacids/H2 blockers and trimethoprim-
sulfamethoxazole for prophylaxis
(1 DS bid)
Anti-emetics before treatment

VAD + verapamil
(40% response)

Response

yes

70–75%

no

Continue as long as
response is achieved;
after maximal response,
give 4 additional cycles
before treatment is
stopped

Third line treatment:
EDAP or α-interferon
3 MU/m^2 3 times a week
or sequential hemibody
irradiation

not
feasible

Investigational
treatment
(including BMT)

Determine
glycoprotein
P-170 (multidrug
resistance protein)

pos

cannot be assayed
or negative

A

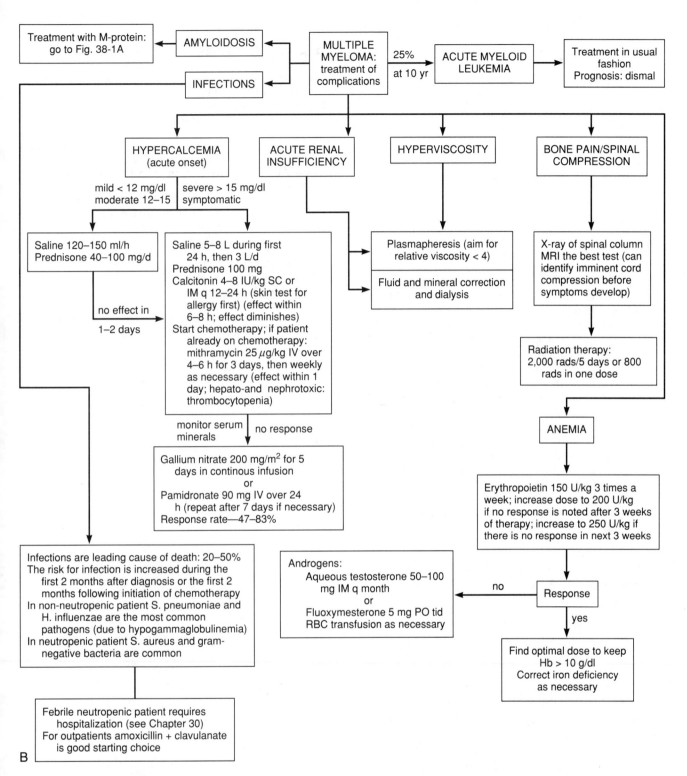

Fig. 38-1 (A and B). **(A)** Treatment of multiple myeloma (MM). An underlying principle of treatment is highly *physiologic* (pharmacologic) through the use of tumorocidal agents. The choice of therapy is based upon *risk/benefit estimates* and the *probability of response* at a particular stage of disease. Note that, for example, a BMT option provides the longest possible survival but also the highest mortality rate (40% five-year survival *vs* 40% treatment-related deaths for allogenic BMT). Follow-up of the patient is also based upon physiologic principles (due to availability of markers that highly correlate with tumor mass—M-protein and β_2-microglobulin). **(B)** An algorithm for special diagnostic/treatment problems in multiple myeloma. (Note that the sequence of choice of antihypercalcemic drugs is a traditional one, with use of recently approved Ga-nitrate and pamidronate at later stage only).

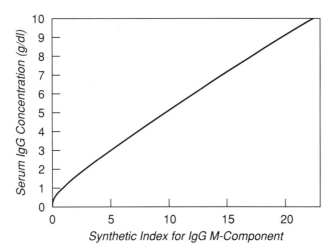

Fig. 38-2. Nomogram for monitoring of treatment effect in multiple myeloma, based upon determination of synthetic index for IgG M-components of subclasses Ig1, IgG2, and IgG4 (which comprise 90% of IgG myelomas). Using the patient's initial serum IgG concentration (g/dl) on the vertical axis, read down from the line to the horizontal axis to determine the synthetic index for that IgG value (Syn1). The same procedure is followed for the follow-up value (Syn2). Syn2/Syn2 × 100 = % of baseline synthetic index and tumor burden. The nomogram is not required for IgG3, IgA, IgD, or IgM serum M-components, and changes in serum values for these Igs can be used directly to determine percent change in tumor burden. (From Salmon and Cassady: Plasma Cell Neoplasms. In DeVita, Hellman S, Rosenberg SA (eds.): Cancer, Principles of Oncology, 3rd Ed. JB Lippincott Co., Philadelphia, 1989, with permission.)

should be determined at frequent intervals (every 2–3 months—see Fig. 38-1 and Fig. 38-2).

Multiple myeloma is *not* a curable disease; however, treatment prolongs survival. The overall median survival is about 2–3 years, but can range from about 15 months (stage IIIB) to 62 months (stage IA). New therapeutic modalities, such as bone marrow transplantation (BMT), therapy with cytokines and antibody against cytokines (e.g., IL-6), and use of agents to overcome resistance, are currently an intensive area of research, but as yet cannot be recommended for use in practice. Recent data on the use of allogenic BMT indicates that this option should be considered in patients younger than 55 years of age after standard treatment has failed. Figures 38-1 A and B show current recommendations for the treatment of multiple myeloma. Figure 38-2 shows nomogram for monitoring treatment effect.

Suggested Readings

Barlogie B: Toward a cure for multiple myeloma? N Engl J Med 325:1304, 1991

Barlogie B, Epstein J, Selvanayagam P, Alexanian R: Plasma cell myeloma: new biological insights and advances in therapy. Blood 73:865, 1989

Bergsagel DE: Use a gentle approach for refractory myeloma patients. J Clin Oncol 6:757, 1988

Buzaid AC, Durie BGM: Management of refractory myeloma. J Clin Oncol 6:889, 1988

Djulbegovic B, Blumenraich M, Joseph G, Hadley T: Melphalan-prednisone *vs* combined therapy in multiple myeloma: a meta-analysis. Blood 78:114a, 1991

Gahrton G, Tura S, Ljungman P, et al.: Allogeneic bone marrow transplantation in multiple myeloma. N Engl J Med 325:1267, 1991

Ludwig H, Fritz E, Kotzmann H, et al.: Erythropoietin treatment of anemia associated with multiple myeloma. N Engl J Med 322:1693, 1990

Malpas JS: New treatments in myeloma: is cure possible? Postgrad Med J 63:425, 1987

39 | Human Immunodeficiency Virus (HIV) Infection

HIV infection is a systemic, immunosuppressive disease caused by the HIV retrovirus. The major routes of HIV infection are sexual activity and blood or blood products. The vast majority of HIV-infected patients, an estimated 1–2 million in the U.S. and 5–10 million worldwide, are asymptomatic. As of October 1991, there were 199,406 registered cases of full-blown symptomatic AIDS (acquired immunodeficiency syndrome) in the U.S. Gay men constitute the largest risk group for AIDS, followed by the IV drug abuser. Only 6% of all U.S. cases are transmitted through heterosexual contact; this mode of transmission is, however, expected to increase as the epidemic matures.

HIV infection is a universally lethal disease. The *natural history* of HIV infection begins with a viral prodrome (mononucleosis-like syndrome), followed by seroconversion, which may take from 3–6 months. Detection of this antibody is a basis for the *diagnosis* of HIV infection (Fig. 39-1). There is a period of latency during which the patient is free of symptoms; the actual duration of this phase is highly variable, with a median duration of 8–10 years. The risk clearly increases over time. In homosexuals, 2% developed AIDS within 2 years of infection, 5% within 3 years, 10% within 4 years, 23% within 6 years, 37% within 8 years, and 48% within 10 years. In hemophiliacs, no cases of AIDS have developed within 2 years of seroconversion, although 22% have developed AIDS within 7 years, with a median time to seroconversion of 36 months.

Several staging systems have been developed to assist in the prediction of the course of HIV infection. Many factors have been identified as important predictors, but there is an overall consensus that the CD4 count is the most important predictor of the course of disease (see box below). This clinical observation is in strong agreement with understanding the pathophysiology of disease—the virus appears to bind specifically to helper (CD4/T4 positive) T cell lymphocytes, causing the acquired immunodeficiency state. This *physiological reasoning* forms a basis for NIH recommendations for clinical management of the HIV infection (Fig. 39-2). This recommendation is coupled with the use of antiretroviral agents such as zidovudine (AZT), and the still largely *probabilistic* estimate that AZT prolongs survival in HIV infection (at least in patients with CD4≤500/mm^3) (Fig. 39-2).

HIV infection can manifest in many acquired hematologic defects, including neutropenia, thrombocytopenia, anemia, and various hematologic malignancies (Fig. 39-3). Overall, once AIDS is developed,

---

Independent Predictors of Developing AIDS

CD4 count ≤200 cell/mm^3

CD4/CD8 (helper/suppressor) ratio ≤25%

Presence of p24 antigen or absence of p24 antibody

β_2-microglobulin ≥3 µg/ml

Data from Cohen et al.: The Aids Knowledge Base, Massachusetts Medical Society, 1990, with permission; note that many factors other than the CD4 count are also identified, but they have not been consistently reproduced in all studies.

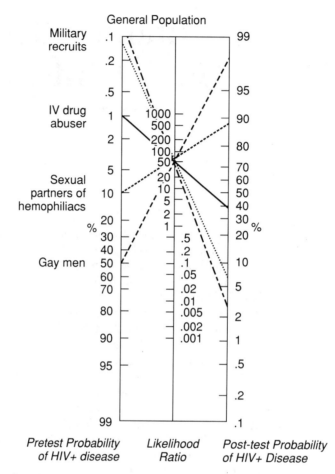

Fig. 39-1. Diagnosis of HIV infection. Sensitivity and specificity of current ELISA tests for detection of antibody against HIV-1 virus is 99.7% and 98.5%, respectively. (LR+ = 66.4, LR− = .003.) (HIV-2 infection is rare in the U.S. and is almost invariably associated with origin or travel to subSaharan Africa.) Only repeatedly positive tests should be considered positive, and they should be confirmed by western blot assay. Note that post-test probability that HIV infection exists should be interpreted in the light of risk factors (pretest probabilities) for HIV infection (results in case of a negative test are not shown for reasons of clarity, but can be easily determined using likelihood ratio figure shown above). (Data of pretest probability estimates taken from Barry: In Panzer RJ, Black ER, Griner PF (eds.): Diagnostic strategies for common medical problems. ACP, Philadelphia, 1990, with permission.) Note also that the risk of transmission of HIV infection from surgeon to patient is 1 in 21 million per hour of surgery if the HIV status of the operator is not known, or 1 in 83,000 per hour of surgery if the surgeon is HIV positive (Data from Lowenfels AB and Wormser G: Risk of transmission of HIV from surgeon to patient. N Engl J Med 325:888, 1991).

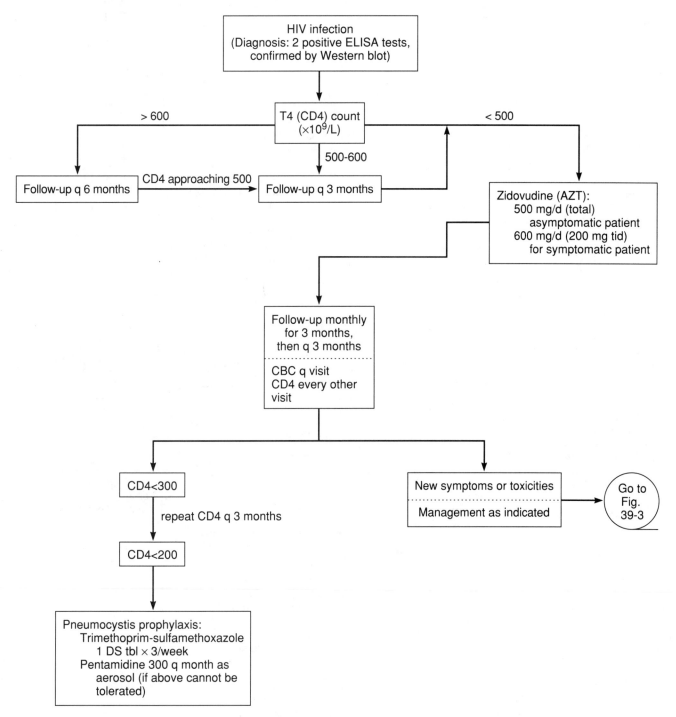

Fig. 39-2. Management of HIV infection. This algorithm is based upon guidelines developed by NIH (Am J Med 89:335, 1990 and recent review article on zidovudine, Can Med Assoc J 143:1177, 1990). Understanding the *pathophysiology* of the disease forms a basis for this recommendation. The use of zidovudine is largely based upon the *probabilistic* evidence that it prolongs survival, and not on evidence that it eradicates infection.

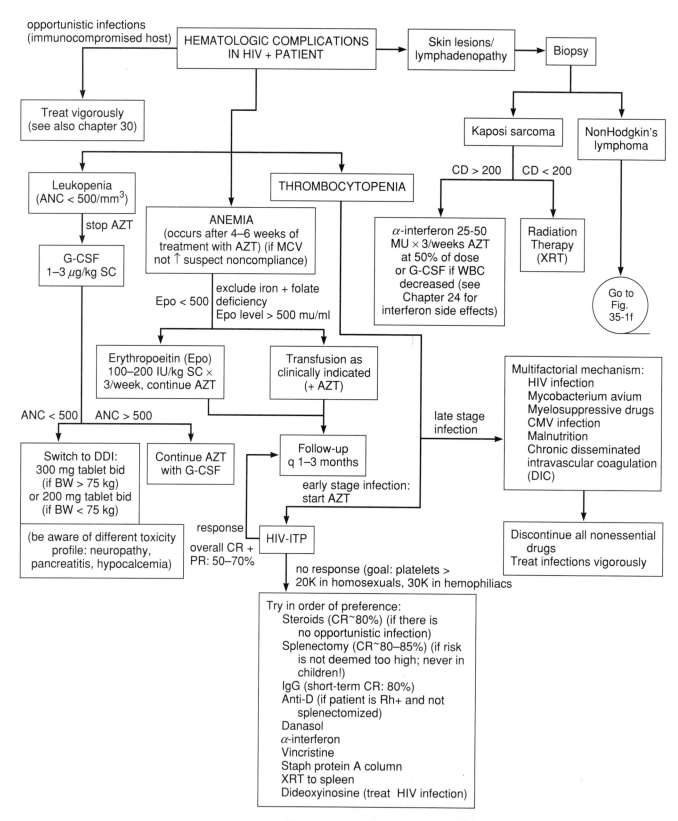

Fig. 39-3. Hematologic complications of HIV infection. This algorithm presents the authors' interpretation of the current literature data. Physiological principles of the fighting of HIV infection, coupled with the institution of various (physiologic) supportive-care maneuvers, dictates the approach to hematologic complications of HIV infection.

the prognosis becomes dismal, with a median survival of treated patients (with AZT) of 770 days and 190 days for untreated patients. Infections (in immunocompromised host) are the major causes of death (see Chapter 30).

Suggested Readings

The Aids Knowledge Base. Cohen PT, Sande MA, Volberding PA (eds.): Massachusetts Medical Society, Waltham, MA, 1990.

Fischl MA, Parker CB, Pettinelli C et al.: A randomized controlled trial of a reduced daily dose of zidovudine in patients with the acquired immunodeficiency syndrome. The AIDS Clinical Trials Group. N Engl J Med 323:1009, 1990

Kimura S, Matsuda J, Ikematsu S et al.: Efficacy of recombinant human granulocyte colony-stimulating factor on neutropenia in patients with AIDS. AIDS 4:1251, 1990

Moore RD, Hidalgo J, Sugland BW: Zidovudine and the natural history of the acquired immunodeficiency syndrome. N Engl J Med 324:1412, 1991

NIH State-of-the-art Conference. State-of-the-art conference on azidothymidine therapy for early HIV infection. Am J Med 89:335, 1990

Rozenbaum W, Gharakhanian S, Navarette MS et al.: Long-term follow-up of 120 patients with AIDS-related Kaposi's sarcoma treated with interferon alpha-2a. J Invest Dermatol 95:161S, 1990

Sloand EM, Pitt E, Chiarello RJ, Nemo GJ: HIV testing. State of the art. JAMA 266:2861, 1991

Walsh CM, Krigel R, Lennette E, Karpatkin S: Thrombocytopenia in homosexual patients: prognosis, response to therapy, and prevalence of antibody to the retrovirus associated with the acquired immunodeficiency syndrome. Ann Intern Med 103:542, 1985

40 Diagnosis of Bleeding Disorders

An optimal diagnostic approach to *bleeding disorders* is based upon the application of *physiologic and probabilistic diagnostic reasoning* (Fig. 40-1), as well as the application of certain *production rules*. The physiologic approach is derived from an understanding of the basic mechanisms of *hemostasis* (too much hemostasis leads to thrombosis, too little hemostasis leads to bleeding). In essence, hemostasis is accomplished by three sequential events: (1) vascular reaction, (2) formation of a platelet plug, and (3) activation of the coagulation cascade. The fourth process of clot lysis follows once the clot is formed. Therefore, a derangement of any of these four processes (i.e., vascular integrity, platelets, coagulation cascade, and clot lysis) leads to bleeding disorders.

What are the diagnostic tests that can help us determine what part of the hemostatic system is affected? A *bleeding history* (see box below) is the most sensitive test one can apply at the outset of the diagnostic workup. If the bleeding history is negative, further workup is not necessary. This relates to *preoperative evaluation* as well. If a bleeding history is positive, the usual practice is to proceed to the ordering of *screening tests*: bleeding time, platelet count, activated partial thromboplastin time (aPTT), prothrombin time (PT), and thrombin time (TT). Table 40-1 shows the relation of diagnostic tests to the physiology of hemostasis and the level of hemostatic elements necessary for normal hemostasis to occur, respectively. The sensitivity and specificity of screening tests are shown in Table 40-2. These tests are sufficiently sensitive that, if they are negative, one may abort any further diagnostic workup

and indicate follow-up only, which is usually the case in current medical practice. This is because the prevalence of *primary hematologic disorders* is so low that, outside of obvious bleeding conditions, false-positive test results will greatly outnumber true-positive results. The pretest probability of bleeding disorders in the general (asymptomatic) population ranges between 0.00017 to 1%, but increases up to 40% in the symptomatic population. Figure 40-2 shows an estimated post-probability of bleeding disorders in these settings (in the sense that "screening" means detection of the disorder in the asymptomatic individual, the term "hemostatic screening tests" should be abandoned).

Screening tests are often not sensitive enough to detect von Willebrand's disease, the most common congenital disorder. They also do not detect rare congenital disorders, such as factor XIII deficiency or α-2-antiplasmin deficiency. A production rule, shown in the box below, should be combined with the algorithms shown in Figure 40-3 in the workup of patients with bleeding disorders.

Acquired bleeding disorders are a much more common cause of abnormal bleeding. In fact, the two most common conditions causing abnormal bleeding are *liver disease* and *disseminated intravascular coagulation (DIC)*.

Figure 40-3 shows an algorithmic approach to the majority of hemostatic disorders. These algorithms assume that a diagnostic workup is indicated and that a bleeding disorder indeed exists. A common practice is to perform parallel testing (i.e., to order a platelet count (CBC), bleeding time (BT) and PT/

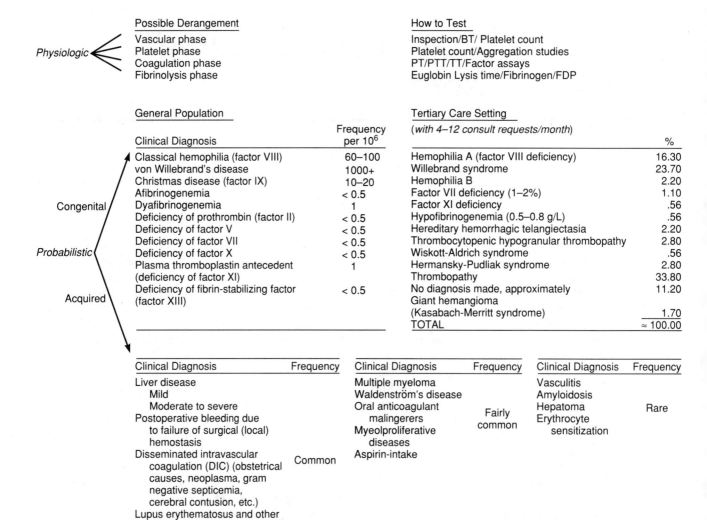

	Possible Derangement	How to Test
Physiologic	Vascular phase	Inspection/BT/ Platelet count
	Platelet phase	Platelet count/Aggregation studies
	Coagulation phase	PT/PTT/TT/Factor assays
	Fibrinolysis phase	Euglobin Lysis time/Fibrinogen/FDP

General Population

Clinical Diagnosis	Frequency per 10^6
Classical hemophilia (factor VIII)	60–100
von Willebrand's disease	1000+
Christmas disease (factor IX)	10–20
Afibrinogenemia	< 0.5
Dyafibrinogenemia	1
Deficiency of prothrombin (factor II)	< 0.5
Deficiency of factor V	< 0.5
Deficiency of factor VII	< 0.5
Deficiency of factor X	< 0.5
Plasma thromboplastin antecedent (deficiency of factor XI)	1
Deficiency of fibrin-stabilizing factor (factor XIII)	< 0.5

Tertiary Care Setting

(with 4–12 consult requests/month)

	%
Hemophilia A (factor VIII deficiency)	16.30
Willebrand syndrome	23.70
Hemophilia B	2.20
Factor VII deficiency (1–2%)	1.10
Factor XI deficiency	.56
Hypofibrinogenemia (0.5–0.8 g/L)	.56
Hereditary hemorrhagic telangiectasia	2.20
Thrombocytopenic hypogranular thrombopathy	2.80
Wiskott-Aldrich syndrome	.56
Hermansky-Pudliak syndrome	2.80
Thrombopathy	33.80
No diagnosis made, approximately	11.20
Giant hemangioma (Kasabach-Merritt syndrome)	1.70
TOTAL	≈ 100.00

Probabilistic — Congenital, Acquired

Clinical Diagnosis	Frequency
Liver disease	
Mild	
Moderate to severe	
Postoperative bleeding due to failure of surgical (local) hemostasis	
Disseminated intravascular coagulation (DIC) (obstetrical causes, neoplasma, gram negative septicemia, cerebral contusion, etc.)	Common
Lupus erythematosus and other immune-diseases, cancer	
Chronic renal disease	

Clinical Diagnosis	Frequency
Multiple myeloma	
Waldenström's disease	
Oral anticoagulant malingerers	Fairly common
Myeolproliferative diseases	
Aspirin-intake	

Clinical Diagnosis	Frequency
Vasculitis	
Amyloidosis	
Hepatoma	Rare
Erythrocyte sensitization	

Fig. 40-1. A conceptual approach to bleeding disorders. An optimal approach combines *physiological, probabilistic* and *deterministic* reasoning strategies (see also Table 40-1).

Preoperative Hemostatic Evaluation[a,b]

History

Have you ever bled for a long time, or developed a swollen tongue or mouth after cutting or biting your tongue, cheek, or lip?

Do you develop bruises larger than a silver dollar without being able to remember when or how you injured yourself? If so, how big was the largest of these bruises?

How many times have you had teeth pulled and what was the longest time that you bled after an extraction? Has bleeding ever started up again the day after an extraction?

What operations have you had, including minor surgeries such as skin biopsies? Was bleeding after surgery ever hard too stop? Have you ever developed unusual bruising in the skin around an area of surgery or injury?

Have you had a medical problem within the past 5 years requiring a doctor's care? If so, what was its nature?

What medication, including aspirin or any other remedies for headaches, colds, menstrual cramps, or other pain, have you taken within the past 7–9 days? Are you currently taking antibiotics or anticoagulants?

Have you ever suffered from liver disease, malnutrition, or diseases of malabsorption?

What is your ethnic/religious background? (Ashkenazic Jews are at higher risk for postoperative bleeding; 11% incidence of factor XI deficiency, usually clinically silent until surgery.)

Has any blood relative had a problem with unusual bruising or bleeding after surgery? Were blood transfusions required to control this bleeding?

Physical Exam

Inspect skin and mucous membranes for petechiae, ecchymoses and hematomas. Look for adenopathy, splenomegaly, and signs of liver disease (hepato-splenomegaly, jaundice, spider naevi).

[a] Data from Rappaport (1983) and Suchman and Grinner (1991).
[b] This preoperative assessment is considered to be superior over hemostatic screening tests for estimate of bleeding risks.

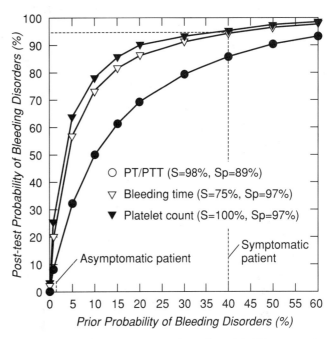

Fig. 40-2. Probability of bleeding disorder if hemostatic screening test(s) are positive. Because of the very low prevalence of bleeding disorders in the asymptomatic population, screening tests offer no advantage over a history and physical exam alone in the excluding of bleeding disorders. In the symptomatic population, post-test probability for bleeding disorders rises dramatically. Recent data, however, suggest that the prevalence of von Willebrand's disease may be as high as 1%. With more realistic operating test characteristics for BT and PTT (see Table 40-2), symptoms alone are still superior to screening tests. (Use Fig. 1-6 to determine individual diagnostic and treatment thresholds.)

Bleeding Disorders: Diagnostic Production Rules

1. *If* the patient is asymptomatic (see box above), *then* a clinical workup for bleeding disorder is not indicated (see Fig. 40-2).

2. *If* the bleeding history is positive and screening tests (BT/PTT/PT/TT) are negative, *then* suspect von Willebrand's disease (vWD) (one negative workup does not exclude vWD).

3. *If* screening tests and workup for vWD and other thrombopathies are negative, *then* test for factor XIII and/or α_2-antiplasmin deficiency (and/or other rare defects of fibrinolytic systems, such as a deficiency of plasminogen activator inhibitor type I).

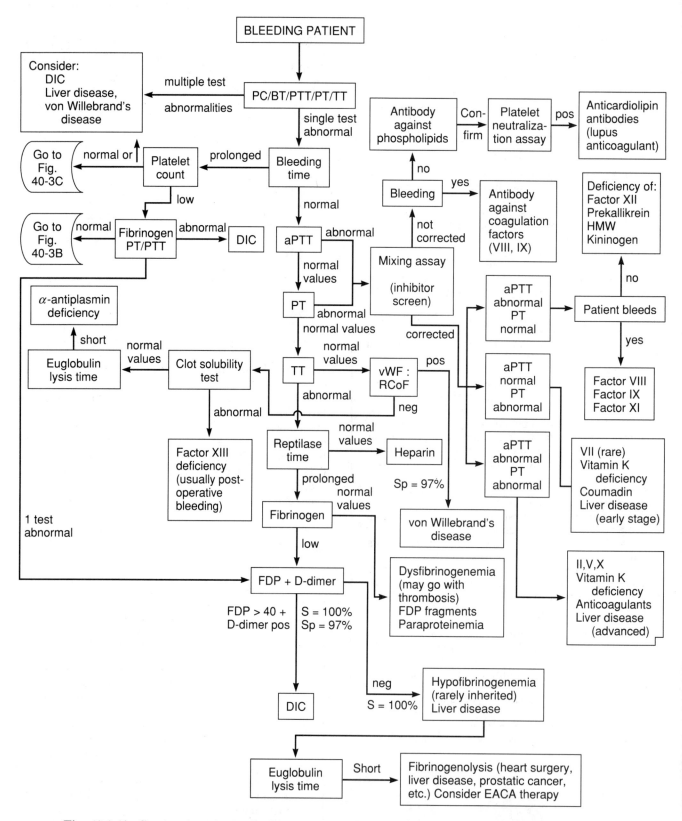

Fig. 40-3 (A–C). An algorithm(s) for diagnosis of bleeding disorders. Their construction is based upon the combination of *physiologic* and *probabilistic* reasoning (see Fig. 40-1). Note that setting alone (principles of *representative heuristic*) can trigger a differential diagnosis (e.g., ICU thrombocytopenia). *Abbreviations*: PC, platelet count; BT, bleeding time; WF: RC/F, von Willebrand factor: ristocetin cofactor assay; RIPA, ristocetin-induced platelet aggregation; vWF:Ag, von Willebrand factor: antigen.

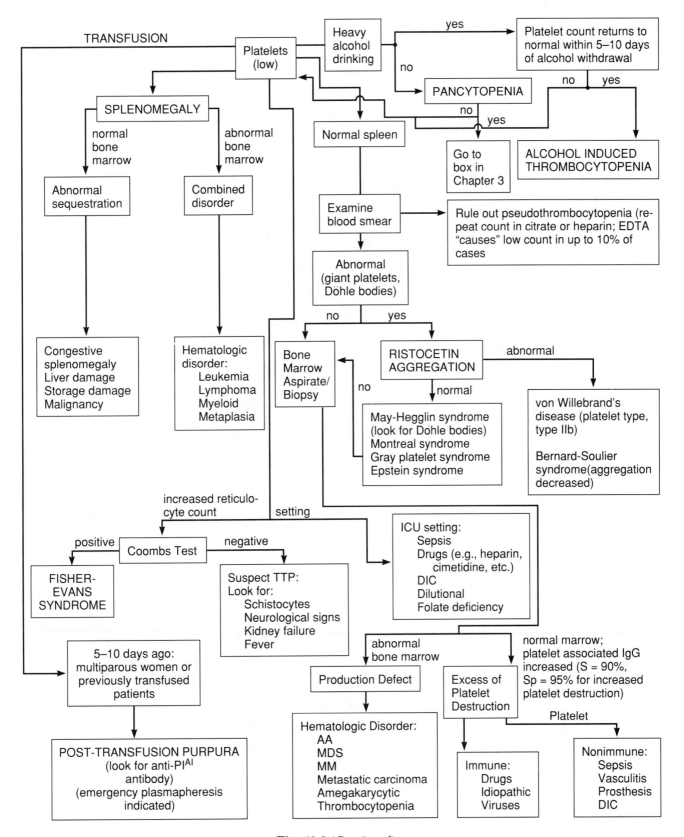

Fig. 40-3 (*Continued*)

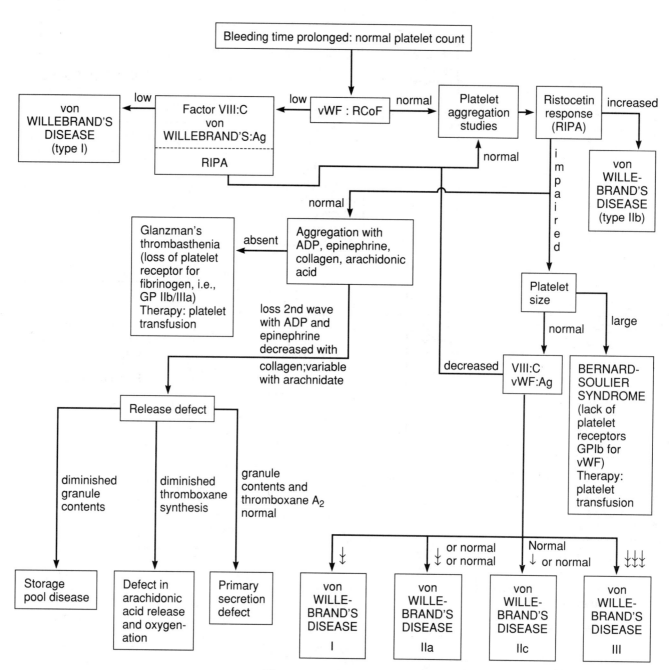

Fig. 40-3 (*Continued*)

Table 40-1. What Hemostatic Tests Actually Test

Diagnostic Test	Hemostatic Area	What is Tested
Inspection	Vascular integrity	Vascular phase
Platelets bleeding time	Primary hemostasis	Quantitative and qualitative platelets defects
aPTT	Intrinsic pathway of coagulation cascade	Deficiencies or inhibitors of: XII, XI, IX, VIII, X, V, II, I
PT	Extrinsic pathway of coagulation cascade	Deficiencies or inhibitors of: VII, X, V, II, I
TT	Final pathway of coagulation cascade	Deficiencies or inhibitors of: IIa, I
Euglobin lysis time	Clot lysis	Rate of clot lysis

Concentration of Hemostatic Elements Needed For Normal Coagulation

Factor	Values Needed For Normal Coagulation
XII	—
XI	20
IX[a]	40
VIII	30
VII[a]	25
X[a]	40
V	40
II[a]	40
I	100 mg/dl
Platelets	>50,000 /μl

[a] Vitamin K dependent factors

Table 40-2. Receiver Operating Characteristic of Hemostatic Screening Tests

Test	Sensitivity (%)	Specificity (%)	Condition
Bleeding time (prolonged)	0–7	96	Postoperative bleeding (asymptomatic patient)
Bleeding time (prolonged)	29–75	88–97	Von Willebrand's disease
Bleeding time (prolonged)	70	80	Thrombocytopenic bleeding
Platelets (decreased)	0–3	92	Postoperative bleeding (asymptomatic patients)
Platelets (decreased)	97–100	97	Thrombocytopenia (theoretical value)
Platelets (decreased)	73–93	48	DIC (Disseminated intravascular coagulation)
aPTT	7–8	90	Postoperative bleeding (low risk)
aPPT	57	67	Postoperative bleeding (high risk)
aPPT	98	89–98	Any intrinsic factor deficiency (<25–40% of normal value)
aPPT	36–60	68–98	Von Willebrand's disease (based on factor VIII deficiency detection)
PT	98–100	89–98	Factor VII deficiency (offers no advantage over history and physical exam in detection of acquired factor VII deficiency associated with liver disease, malnutrition or malabsorption)
TT	0–5	97	Postoperative bleeding (asymptomatic)
TT	20–50	80–90	Low fibrinogen (estimate based upon measurements in DIC)
Euglobin lysis time	?	?	Largely abandoned test: time-consuming, poor sensitivity and specificity

PTT/TT at the same time). Further workup will depend on which test(s) is abnormal. Conditions are identified as the workup is pursued.

Suggested Readings

Bachmann F: Diagnostic approach to mild bleeding disorders. Semin Hematol 17:292, 1980

Day HJ, Rao KA: Evaluation of platelet function. Semin Hematol 23:89, 1986

Lind SE: The bleeding time does not predict surgical bleeding. Blood 77:3547, 1991

Rapaport SI: Preoperative hemostatic evaluation: which tests, if any? Blood 61:229, 1983

Rodgers RP, Levin J: A critical reappraisal of bleeding time. Semin Thromb Hemost 16:1, 1990

Rohrer MJ, Michelotti MC, Nahrwold DL: A prospective evaluation of the efficacy of preoperative coagulation testing. Ann Surg 208:554, 1988

Suchman AL, Griner PF: Diagnostic use of the activated partial thromboplastin time and prothrombin time. Ann Intern Med 104:810, 1986

Suchman AL, Griner PF: Coagulation disorders. In Panzer RJ, Black ER, Griner PF (eds.): Diagnostic strategies for common medical problems. American College of Physicians, Philadelphia 1991

Chronic Idiopathic (Autoimmune) Thrombocytopenic Purpura

41

Chronic idiopathic (autoimmune) thrombocytopenic purpura (ITP) is a relatively common hematologic problem, and the most common autoimmune disorder in women of childbearing age. This is predominantly a disease of the adult population, contrary to acute ITP. The overall incidence of thrombocytopenia is estimated to be 4.5 and 7.5 per 100,000 patients for males and females, respectively. An approximated 50% of these patients will have ITP. The diagnosis of ITP is still a diagnosis of exclusion. A "Coombs test" for antibodies against platelets is not only cumbersome and time-consuming, but has many false-positive and false-negative results. An interesting analogy regarding this test was recently proposed: the increase of total platelet IgG (TPlIgG) in patients with thrombocytopenia is equivalent to the reticulocyte counts in the evaluation of patients with anemia; measurements of surface IgG (antiplatelet antibodies) (SIgG) could be considered equivalent to a real Coombs test to detect antiRBC antibodies in autoimmune hemolytic anemia. Sensitivity and specificity of TPlIgG in distinguishing between immune *vs* nonimmune causes of thrombocytopenia is between 84–90% and 95–97%, respectively.

The treatment of chronic ITP generally relates to three different clinical situations (Fig. 41-1): (1) treatment of life-threatening disease, (2) typical chronic ITP, and (3) chronic ITP in pregnancy. Hospitalization and urgent treatment is required in patients with platelet counts of less than 5,000 to 10,000/mm^3 (5.0–10.0 $\times$ 10^9/L), excessive or central nervous system (CNS) bleeding. The cornerstone of therapy is still steroids, followed by a splenectomy and high doses of IV IgG. A variety of other treatments are still experimental, not as effective, or too toxic to be used as a first-line treatment. Long-term remission after steroids is probably around 10–30%, and after splenectomy, about 60%. Additional partial remission can be expected in about 10–20% in both treatment regimens. The overall mortality rate in chronic ITP is less than 5%, but can be as high as 16% in the group of patients refractory to both steroids and splenectomy. In addition, those individuals older than 60 years and those with a previous history of bleeding are at major risk for severe hemorrhages in ITP. In general, severe bleeding episodes do not occur at platelet counts $\geq$ 30 $\times$ 10^9/L.

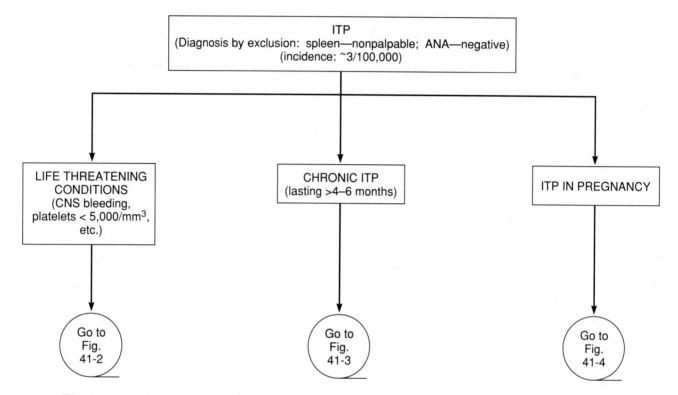

Fig. 41-1. Treatment of chronic idiopathic (autoimmune) thrombocytopenic purpura (ITP). Management is dependent on the clinical setting. The element of time (chronic *vs* emergency) and estimates of the risk/benefit dominate clinical strategies of management of ITP.

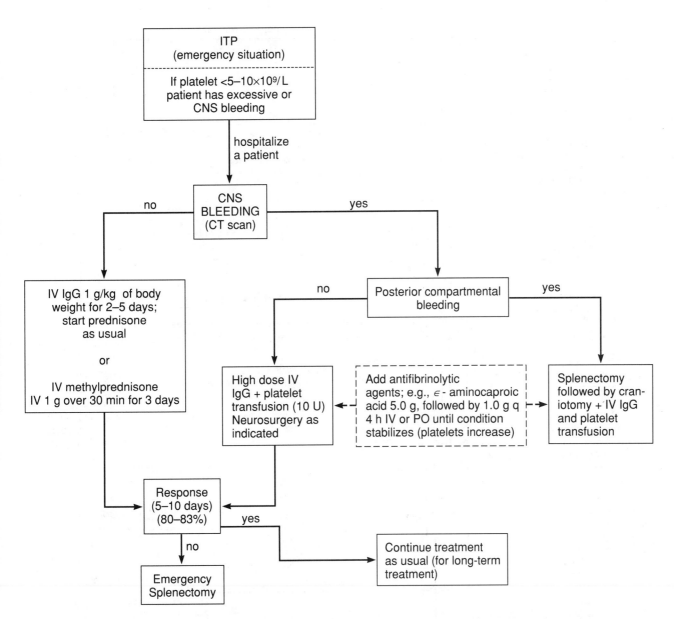

Fig. 41-2. Treatment of ITP in emergency situations. The major risk is CNS bleeding. The most important risk factors are age (>60) and previous history of bleeding. Note that severe bleeding virtually does not exist if platelets are > 30.000/mm³. In life-threatening situations, the decision making strategy is usually to *"throw" all available options* ("an event you can't afford to have happen"; the strategy with highest benefit/risk ratio). Although not tested, there are some reports (Arch Intern Med 149:1959, 1989) that antifibrinolytic agents may be useful in the treatment of dangerous thrombocytopenia. (Broken arrow denotes alternative strategy.)

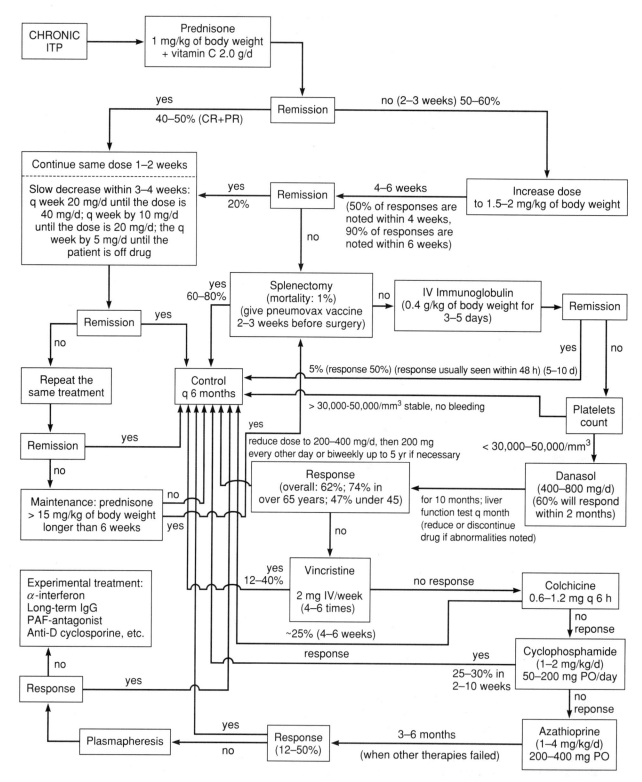

Fig. 41-3. Long-term therapy of ITP. This sequence of treatments is based upon the estimate of the *probability of response and risks* associated with each treatment. There is a general consensus regarding the two first choices of management options (steroids and splenectomy). The order of the use of other options is not well-established, and is represented here by these authors' experience and literature estimates. Note that the majority of authors do not consider high-dose IgG an option in long-term treatment of chronic ITP. However, we have seen some long-term responses and, given the rarity of serious side effects (and despite high cost), it is included in our algorithm. Also, note that therapy with anti-D antibody is not effective in splenectomized and non-Rh positive patients.

198

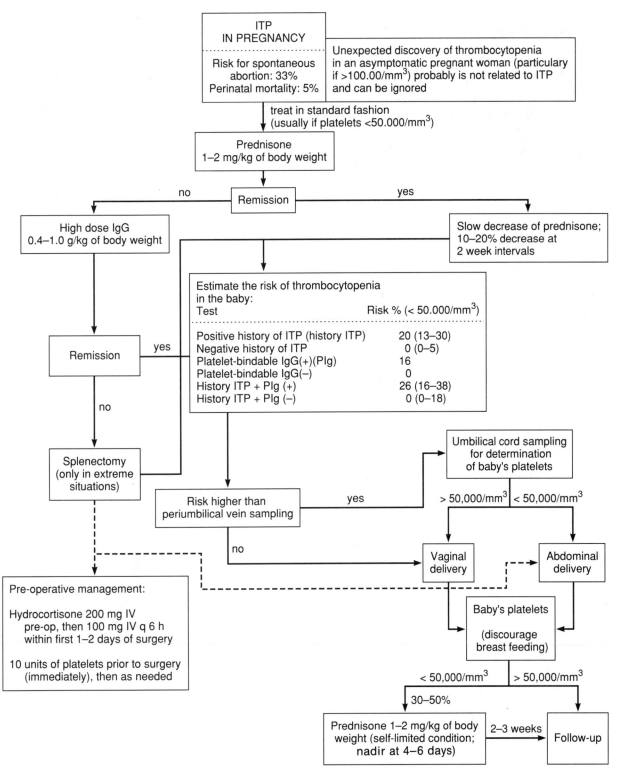

Fig. 41-4. Management of ITP in pregnancy will depend on the *estimates of the risk of thrombocytopenia in the baby* (Risk estimate taken from: Samuels et al.: N Engl J Med 323:229, 1990), as well as on the local expertise of platelet determination in the umbilical vein sample. Note that there are authors who advocate that the management of ITP in pregnancy should not differ from the standard approach. Others would prefer the use of high IgG during pregnancy to avoid steroid side effects, but would also avoid periumbilical vein sampling and perform a cesarean section only according to obstetric indications. (Broken arrows denote alternative strategies.)

Suggested Readings

Ahn YS, Rocha R, Mylvaganam R, et al.: Long-term danazol therapy in autoimmune thrombocytopenia: unmaintained remission and age-dependent response in women. Ann Intern Med 111:723, 1989

Berchtold P, McMillan R: Therapy of chronic thrombocytopenia purpura in adults. Blood 74:2309, 1989

Burrows RF, Kelton JG: Incidentally detected thrombocytopenia in healthy mothers and their infants. N Engl J Med 319:142, 1988

Cortelazzo S, Finazzi G, Buelli M, et al.: High risk of severe bleeding in aged patients with chronic idiopathic thrombocytopenic purpura. Blood 77:31, 1991

Martin JN, Morrison JC, Files JC: Autoimmune thrombocytopenic purpura: current concepts and recommended practices. Am J Obstet Gynecol 150:86, 1984

42 | Hemophilia A and B

Hemophilia A and *B* are X-linked recessive disorders that occur almost exclusively in males. These types of hemophilia comprise about 97% of all congenital coagulation abnormalities. The prevalence of classic hemophilia is between 60–100 per million population, and that of Christmas disease about 10–20 per million population. In about 30–50% of cases, no positive family history exists (i.e., a new mutation occurs). These patients show typical *coagulation type bleeding*: deep, large intramuscular bruises and hematomas, usually occurring late (1–4 hours) after trauma. Postoperative and dental bleeding typically occur late—hours or even days after the procedure. The most common bleeding occurs in the joints (75% of all bleeding episodes—order of decreasing frequency: knees, elbows, ankles, shoulders, wrists, hips) and in subcutaneous tissue and muscles (calf, thigh, buttocks, forearm). Hematuria occurs very frequently in severe hemophiliacs, and epistaxis is quite common in childhood. Gastrointestinal bleeding is rare outside the existence of structural abnormalities. Bleeding in hemophiliacs is in sharp contrast to the purpuric type of bleeding seen in thrombocytopenia and von Willebrand's disease, which starts immediately after trauma and is often controlled by pressure. Epistaxis and gastrointestinal bleeding are often major sources of bleeding in these diseases (see Chapter 43).

The *diagnosis* of hemophiliac conditions is easy; most patients will have a prolonged PTT, with other screening hemostatic tests being normal. The PTT test is sensitive enough to detect procoagulant levels below 25%. A specific diagnosis is made by assaying the level of factor VIII or IX. The diagnosis is fol-lowed by the *estimation of the severity of disease*: mild (with 6–50% factor level), moderate (with factor level between 2–5%), and severe (with factor level ≤1%). About two-thirds of all patients will have moderate to severe disease.

Principles of *treatment* follow *physiological lines of reasoning*: replacement therapy with general measures (avoidance of aspirin and related compounds, IM injections, etc.) against whatever might compromise good hemostasis. Dosages are calculated according to which type of bleeding (mild *vs* moderate *vs* severe) is occurring. The treatment schedule depends on the half-life of the factors: 8–12 hours for factor VIII and 18–24 hours for factor IX (see Fig. 42-1 for details of hemophilia management). *Major problems* in the treatment of hemophilia are the *development of inhibitors* (see Chapter 44 for treatment of hemophilia patients with inhibitors) and *transmission of viral disease* (hepatitis B, C, and AIDS) by factor concentrates. Before the advent of heat-treated concentrates, 90–100% of patients had elevated transaminase or developed antibody against HBsAg. So far, about 1,000 cases of AIDS have been reported among hemophiliacs, and about 70% of patients treated with concentrates before 1984 are HIV positive. No seroconversion has been reported since 1985. New concentrates appear to be viral-inactivated (*Note*—cryoprecipitate is *less* safe than commercial products). Since the benefits of many factor concentrates seem to be the same, their cost is becoming the major issue in choice of concentrate. It is believed that pasteurized or monoclonally purified products are currently the products of choice for treatment of new hemophiliacs of those who are HIV

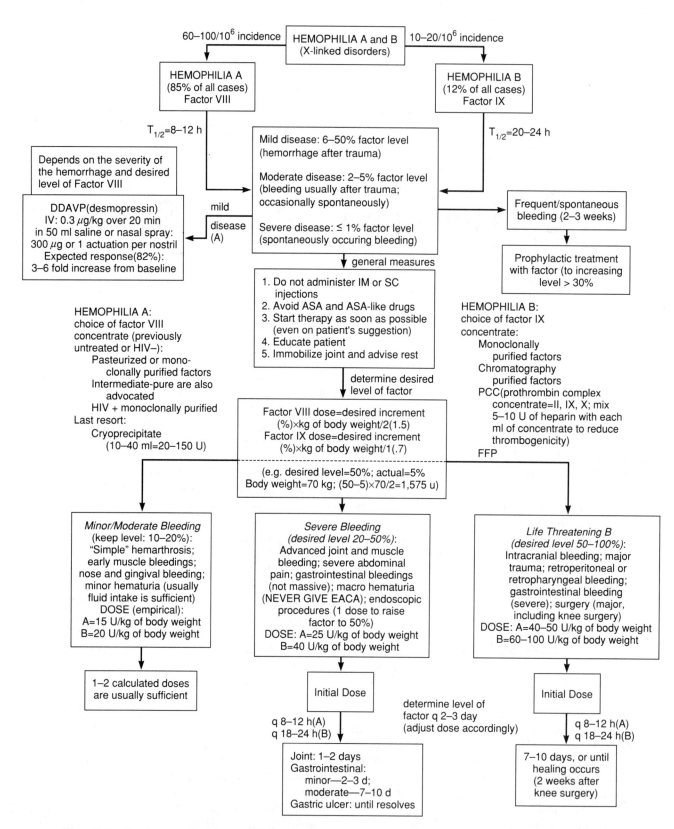

Fig. 42-1. Treatment of patients with hemophilia A and B. The *physiological line of reasoning* is the dominating strategy in management of these patients. This consists of replacement of the deficient factor; determination of the dosage is based upon the existence of a direct correlation between the number of bleeding episodes and the factor(s) level and pharmacokinetics of factor(s) concentrate. *Cost/effectiveness* estimate plays a major role in choice of particular factor concentrate.

Table 42-1. Comparison of Factor VIII and Factor IX Products[a]

Intermediate Purity and High Purity Factor VIII Products Derived From Human Plasma[a]

Product Name	Manufacturer	Method of Inactivation	Hepatitis Safety Studies in Humans	
			With This Product	With Another Product But Similar Method
Profilate OSD	Alpha	Solvent-detergent, 27°C, 6 hours	No	
Koate-HP	Cutter	Solvent-detergent, 27°C, 6 hours	No	
NY Blood Center FVIII-SD	NYBC	Solvent-detergent, ≥ 24°C, 6 hours	Yes	
Humate-P	Behringwerke (distributed by Armour)	Heated in solution (pasteurized) 60°C, 10 hours	Yes	
Melate	NYBC	Solvent-detergent, ≥ 24°C, 6 hours	No	

Immunoaffinity Purified Factor VIII Products (Ultrapure Products) Derived From Human Plasma

Monoclate P	Armour	Pasteurized, 60°C, 10 hours	Yes (ongoing)	Yes
Hemofil M	Baxter-Hyland	Solvent-detergent ≥ 25°C, ≥ 10 hours	Yes	
Coagulation f.VIII Method M	(Manufactured by Baxter-Hyland for American Red Cross)	Solvent-detergent, ≥ 25°C, ≥ 10 hours	No	Yes

Porcine Factor VIII

Hyate C	Porton Products, Ltd.	No viral inactivation, but polyelectrolyte chromatography purification	Yes	

Factor IX Products Licensed in the U.S.
Factor IX Complex Concentrates

Konyne HT	Cutter	Dry heat, 68°C, 72 hours	No	No
Konyne 80	Cutter	Dry heat, 80°C 72 hours	No	Yes
Proplex T	Baxter-Hyland	Dry heat, 68°C, 144 hours	No	No
Profilnine HT (wet method)	Alpha	Heated in N-Heptane solution 60°C, 20 hours	No	Yes (with HCV transmission)

Coagulation Factor IX Products[b]

AlphaNine	Alpha	Heated in N-Heptane solution 60°C, 20 hours	No	Yes

Activated Factor IX Complex Concentrates

Autoplex	Baxter-Hyland	Dryheat, 68°C, 144 hours	No	No
FEIBA	Immuno	Vapor heated (10 hours, 60°C 1190 mbar plus 1 hour, 80°C, 1375 mbar)	No	Yes

[a] December 1991
[b] Mononine, monoclonal-purified factor IX—license pending.
(Source: National Hemophilia Foundation Information Exchange.)

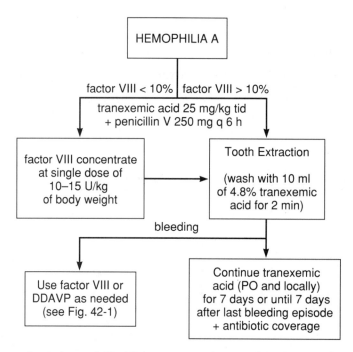

Fig. 42-2. Tooth extraction in hemophilia. This recommendation is based upon a Swedish protocol (Data from Lancet II:566, 1988). Standard textbooks, however, recommend raising administering factor to 50% (25 IU/kg) preoperatively (single dose) and to start tranexemic acid, 500 mg tid or ε-aminocaproic acid 4.0 g every 4 hours for 10 days. The postoperative pain is easily controlled with acetaminophen.

negative. For HIV-positive patients, concentrates that are viral-inactive and highly purified are recommended, for it is believed that by further reduction in the extraneous protein overload, immune function may improve and HIV infection may slow down.

With the introduction of replacement therapy in the 1960s and comprehensive home programs, there have been significant reductions in morbidity (>50%) and mortality for hemophiliacs. (See Table 42-1 for comparison of currently available concentrates in the U.S.) Life expectancy has approached normal. However, diseases due to viral transmission (hepatitis B, C, and AIDS) significantly reduce life expectancy in some patients. It is estimated that about 20% of patients will develop chronic liver disease and cirrhosis. The median life expectancy of 68 years in the decade from 1971–1980 declined to only 49 in the decade from 1981–1990, largely due to HIV infection. However, with the advent of new recombinant factors, this problem is expected to be eliminated. Figures 42-1 and 42-2 depict details of the clinical management of patients suffering from hemophilia.

Suggested Readings

Biasi Rd, Rocino A, Miraglia E, Mastrullo L, Quirino AA: The impact of a very high purity factor VIII concentrate on the immune system of human immunodeficiency virus-infected hemophiliacs: a randomized, prospective, two-year comparison with an intermediate purity concentrate. Blood 78:1919, 1991

Brettler DB, Levine PH: Factor concentrates for treatment of hemophilia: which one to choose? Blood 73:2067, 1989

Goedert JJ, Kessler CM, Aledort LM, et al: A prospective study of human immunodeficiency virus type 1 infection and the development of AIDS in subjects with hemophilia. N Engl J Med 321:1141, 1989

Jones PK, Ratnoff OD: The changing prognosis of classic hemophilia (factor VIII "deficiency"). Ann Intern Med 114:641, 1991

Kim HC, McMillan CW, White CG, Bergman GE: Clinical experience of a new monoclonal antibody purified factor IX: half-life, recovery, and safety in patients with hemophilia B. Semin Hematol 27:30, 1990

Pederson SS, Ingerslev J, Ramstrom G, Blomback M: Management of oral bleeding in haemophilic patients. Lancet ii:566, 1988

Smith KJ, Lusher JM, Cohen AR, Salzman P: Initial experience with a new pasteurized monoclonal antibody purified factor VIIIC. Semin Hematol 27:25, 1990

43 | Von Willebrand's Disease

Von Willebrand's disease (vWD) is the most common hereditary bleeding disorder; prevalence of this disease may be as high as 1% (0.57%–1.15%). The disease is characterized by a reduction in the von Willebrand's factor (vWF) levels in plasma and tissues or by a qualitative defect in the vWF. Though acquired vWD is also described in the literature (usually within a setting of myeloproliferative disorders), this disease is inherited in the great majority of cases in autosomal dominant fashion. There are numerous subtypes of vWD, but more than 70% of cases are type I. *Mucocutaneous bleeding* is the most common symptom in these patients, with 60% showing epistaxis, 40% easy bruising and hematomas, 35% menorrhagia, and 35% gingival bleeding. Gastrointestinal bleeding occurs in about 10% of patients, about 35% report bleeding after dental procedures, 25% report postpartum bleeding, and 20% report postoperative bleeding. Clinical symptoms in mild or moderate disease usually ameliorate by the second or third decade of life. Death from bleeding occurs rarely.

A *diagnosis* is established by the determination of the level of factor VIII:C and factor vWF:Ag (Ag = antigen), bleeding time, ristocetin cofactor assay (vWF:RCoF), and platelet aggregation with ristocetin (RIPA) (see also Table 43-1 for operating test characteristics in diagnosis of vWD). It can be noted that, by and large, these tests suffer from low sensitivity, and therefore *results from a single de-termination do not rule out a diagnosis of vWD.* vWF:RCoF is considered the gold standard test, although precise classification may be obtained only by an analysis of multimers of von Willebrand's heterogenous protein, using techniques of crossed immunoelectrophoresis (CIE) and SDS-polyacrylamide gel electrophoresis (see Table 43-2).

For practical purposes, it is important to distinguish between type I, type IIb, other types of II, and type III disease. Based upon this distinction, *therapy* is chosen. Desmopressin (DDAVP) is the treatment of choice in type I, cryoprecipitate is used in type II disease (DDAVP can cause hyperaggregation of platelets in type IIb, with subsequent thrombocytopenia, and therefore is considered contraindicated in type IIB and platelet type of disease), and cryoprecipitate + DDAVP may be used in type III disease. Figure 43-1 shows details of the treatment of vWD with typical response dynamics. Cryoprecipitate, once considered the treatment of choice in therapy for all types of vWD, has gradually been replaced by DDAVP and recently by *intermediate purity concentrates*, which are rich in high-molecular-weight vWF multimers (Humate-P concentrate seems to be the richest one available on the U.S. market today), and which appear to carry no risk for transmission of viral diseases, as does cryoprecipitate. Figure 43-2 shows recommendations for the treatment of vWD in the surgical setting.

Table 43-1. Operating Characteristics of Common Tests Used in Diagnosis of von Willebrand's Disease

Test	Sensitivity (%)	Specificity (%)
Symptoms alone	52	76
Bleeding time	29–75	88–97
Factor VIII:C	37–59	77–97
vWF:Ag	53–81	97
vWF:RCoF	50–72	97
RIPA	52	93–97

(Data from Lian and Deykin: Am J Med 60:344, 1976, and Miller et al.: Blood 54:117, 1979.)

Table 43-2. Characteristic Features of Various Types of von Willebrand's Disease

Feature	Type I	Type IIA	Type IIB	Platelet Type	Type IIC	Type III
Genetic transmission	Autosomal dominant	Autosomal dominant	Autosomal dominant	Autosomal dominant	Autosomal recessive	Autosomal recessive, homozygous, or doubly heterozygous
Plate count	Normal	Normal	Normal or decreased	Low normal or decreased	Normal	Normal
Bleeding time	Prolonged or normal	Prolonged	Prolonged	Prolonged	Prolonged	Prolonged
Factor VIII:C	Decreased or normal	Decreased or normal	Decreased or normal	Normal or decreased	Normal	Substantially decreased
vWF:Ag	Decreased	Decreased or normal	Decreased or normal	Normal or decreased	Decreased or normal	Absent or minute amounts
vWF:RCoF	Decreased	Substantially decreased	Decreased or normal	Decreased or normal	Decreased	Absent
RIPA	Decreased or normal	Absent or decreased	Increased	Increased	Decreased	Absent
CIE	Normal	Abnormal	Abnormal	Abnormal	Abnormal double peak	Variable—usually abnormal
Plasma SDS multimers	All multimers present; may have decreased HMW multimers	Large and intermediate forms absent	Large multimers absent	Large multimers absent	Large multimers absent; doublet multimer structure	Variable to absent
Platelet SDS multimers	As above for plasma	Large and intermediate forms absent (quantity of VWF:Ag normal)	Normal multimers in platelets (quantity normal)	Normal	Large multimers absent; doublet multimer structure	Absent
Response to desmopressin	Hemostasis restored to normal	Although factor vWF:Ag increases, multimeric abnormality is not corrected	Transient correction of multimeric abnormality; possible correction of bleeding time; decreased platelet count	Transient correction of multimeric abnormality; decreased platelet count		No response
Possible pathogenesis	Abnormal release from sites of synthesis	Inability to form or stabilize large multimers	Intrinsic abnormality of vWF increases tissue binding	Abnormality of platelet membrane (GP Ib-IX)	Intrinsic abnormality with doublet structure	Reduced synthesis or rapid breakdown at sites of synthesis

Abbreviations: Ag, antigen; C, procoagulant activity; CIE, crossed immunoelectrophoresis; GP, glycoprotein; HMW, high-molecular-weight; RCoF, ristocetin cofactor; RIPA, ristocetin-induced platelet aggregation; SDS, sodium dodecyl sulfate; vWF, von Willebrand factor.
(From Triplett DA: Mayo Clin Proc 66:832, 1991, with permission.)

von WILLEBRAND'S
DISEASE
(avoid nonsteroidal anti-inflammatory
drugs (NSAIDS); give acetaminophen
for pain control; ask patient about
previous response to the therapy)

goal of treatment:
a – to increase factor VIII:C to hemostatic levels (see hemophilia chapter)
b – to increase vWF:RCoF >50% and correct bleeding time (if possible)

Type
I

Type
IIb

Type
IIa, IIc

Type
III

DDAVP 0.3 μg/kg in
saline infusion
over 20–30 min IV (qd or
bid) (or spray
150 μg/ nostril)

Humate-P 30–50 U/kg q
8–12 h or cryoprecipitate
1–2 bags/10 kg of
body weight q 8–12 h
DDAVP contraindicated!

Humate-P 30–50 U/kg q
8–12 h or cryoprecipitate
1–2 bags/10 kg of
body weight q 8–12 h

Humate-P 30–50 U/kg q
8–12 h or cryoprecipitate
1–2 bags/10 kg of
body weight q 8–12 h
+DDAVP after infusion

increases factor VIII:C
and vWF 3x (2–10 fold)

(300 μg of spray=0.2 μg/kg
of IV dose)

add Humate-P/Cryo if
bleeding continues

Continue until bleeding
stops; bleeding time is
best test to monitor treatment
effect (usually corrects within
4–6 hours)

Factor VIIIC continue to rise
within 24–48 h; VIIIR:Ag and
VIIIR:Co have $T_{1/2}$ = 4–6 h

Specific Bleeding Problems:

Epistaxis:
    Tranexemic acid 1–2 g tid or
    ϵ-aminocaproic acid 2–6 g qid + local measures (e.g.,
    microfibrillar collagen strips)

Severe menorrhagia:
    Humate-P + high dose conjugated estrogen (40 mg q
    4 h IV for up to 6 doses) + estrogen-progestin tablets
    (with 5 mg progestin) (give 2 tablets initially, then 1
    tablet qid; taper according to the response) (less severe
    menorrhagia can be treated with oral contraceptives only)

Pregnancy:
    Give Humate-P/Cryo if factor VIII:C<30% or DDAVP in
    type I (likelihood of the bleeding is minimal if factor
    VIII:C>50%)
    Most deliveries can be vaginal

Alloantibody to vWF:
    Avoid replacement products containing vWF
    (danger of anamnestic reaction); try DDAVP
    or pure Factor VIII:C in hemophilia type of bleeding

Autoantibody to vWF:
    Treat underlying cause (myeloproliferative diseases,
    connective tissue diseases, etc.)
    DDAVP in mild cases;
    Humate-P/Cryo → if no response try following:
        IgG 1.0 g/kg of body weight × 2
        Steroids
        Porcine factor VIII (40 U/kg)
        Protein A column with plasmapheresis followed by
            Humate-P/Cryo
        Prothrombin complex concentrate (e.g., FEIBA)
        Splenectomy (e.g., in hairy cell leukemia)

Fig. 43-1. Treatment of von Willebrand's disease. The *physiological strategy* (replacement therapy of deficient material) is largely supplemented by an estimate of the *probability of the response* to the particular treatment maneuver. Avoidance of unnecessary risk of viral transmission makes cryoprecipitate a last treatment option.

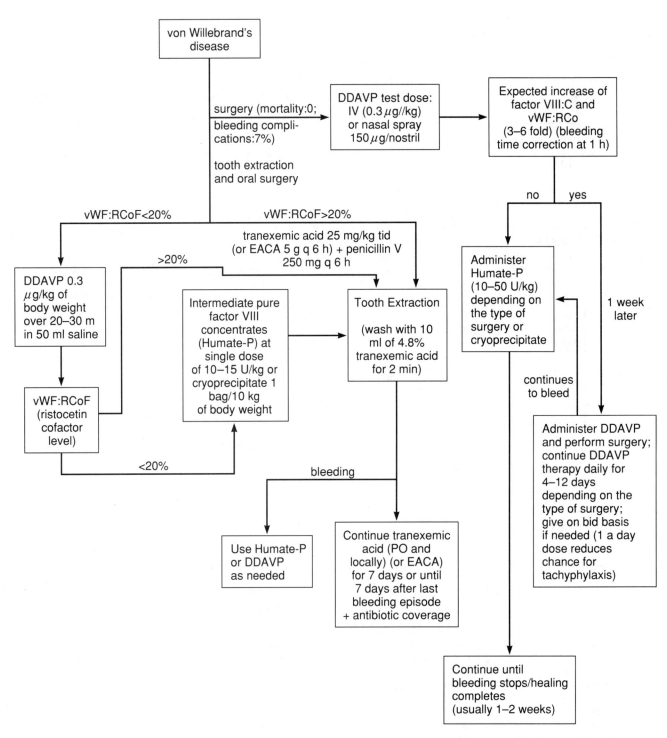

Fig. 43-2. Surgery in von Willebrand's disease. Data for protocol for oral surgery from Sindet-Pederson, et al., Lancet ii:566, 1988).

Suggested Readings

Aledort LM: Treatment of von Willebrand's disease. Mayo Clin Proc 66:841, 1991

Blomback M, Johansson G, Johnsson H, et al.: Surgery in patients with von Willebrand's disease. Br J Surg 76:398, 1989

Bowie EJW: Von Willebrand's disease. Clinical picture, diagnosis, and treatment. Clin Lab Med 4:303, 1984

Cattaneo M, Moia M, Valle DP, et al.: DDAVP shortens the prolonged bleeding times of patients with severe von Willebrand's disease treated with cryoprecipitate. Evidence for a mechanism action independent of released von Willebrand factor. Blood 74:1972, 1989

de la Fuente B, Kasper K, Rickles FR, Hoyer W: Response of patients with mild and moderate hemophilia A and von Willebrand's disease to treatment with desmopressin. Ann Intern Med 103:6, 1985

Logan LJ: Management of von Willebrand's disease. Prog Clin Biol Res 324:279, 1990

Rodeghiero F, Castman G, Dini E: Epidemiological investigation of the prevalence of von Willebrand's disease. Blood 69:454, 1987

Triplett DA: Laboratory diagnosis of von Willebrand's Disease. Mayo Clin Proc 66:832, 1991

44 Acquired Anticoagulants (Inhibitors)

In general, *anticoagulants (inhibitors)* are antibodies that may be directed against specific coagulation proteins (associated with an increased risk of *hemorrhage*) or against *negatively charged phospholipids*. Interestingly, although antibodies against phospholipids are a common cause of prolonged PTT and PT, they appear to be associated with an increased risk of thrombosis.

Inhibitors are described in the literature against almost all coagulation factors, but they are by far most frequently directed against factor VIII and IX, and occur in both the hemophilic and nonhemophilic population. It is estimated that about 6–8% of patients with hemophilia A will develop inhibitors, with the prevalence of inhibitors against factor IX somewhat less. Incidence of acquired hemophilia in the general population is about 0.2–1 per million per annum. In hemophiliacs these inhibitors are *alloantibodies*, and in almost all cases are IgG immunoglobulins (IgG4 predominates). Nonhemophilic patients develop *autoantibodies*, usually within the setting of rheumatoid arthritis, malignancies, drug reactions, etc., but they may occur in older patients with no underlying problems (in about 46% of cases) or in peripartum women (8%).

A *production rule* may be of diagnostic help: *If* a patient with hemophilia responds suboptimally to treatment, or a nonhemophilic (usually older) patient suddenly shows symptoms and signs of bleeding diathesis, *then* suspect inhibitor(s). It is usually diagnosed after a prolonged aPTT is found. The first evidence that circulating anticoagulant is present may be obtained with a "50:50 mix" of the patient's plasma with a normal plasma. While in deficiency states, aPTT will be corrected on the mixture with normal plasma; this will not be the case if the patient has developed an inhibitor. (A value of ≤4 sec is considered correction, and a difference ≥7 sec between normal plasma and that of a mixture of normal and patient's plasma is taken as strong evidence for inhibitory activity; at the same time, specific factors against which the inhibitor is developed will be consistently *low*, e.g., factor VIII).

Treatment of the patient with an inhibitor is difficult. Fig. 44-1 shows an algorithm for management of the patient with an inhibitor against factor VIII. Treatment is individualized according to the type of antibody (autoantibody *vs* alloantibody), the level of inhibitors, and is dependent upon the patient's anamnestic response to factor VIII infusion (low responder *vs* high responders). Patients with inhibitors to factor IX are usually treated with the same material (factor IX, PCC) as usual. Immunosuppressive therapy is much more effective in patients with autoantibodies than in those with alloantibodies (hemophiliacs).

The *prognosis* is worse for nonhemophilic patients. Major bleeding occurs in about 87% of patients, with the death rate for these patients exceeding 20%. In hemophiliacs, the presence of inhibitors does not appear to significantly alter life expectancy.

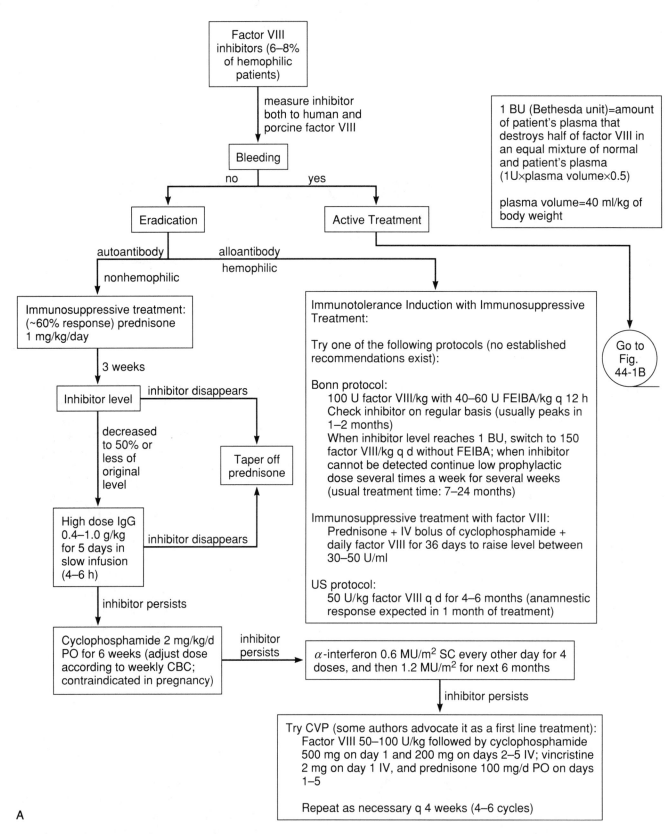

Factor VIII
inhibitors (6–8%
of hemophilic
patients)

measure inhibitor
both to human and
porcine factor VIII

Bleeding

no — yes

1 BU (Bethesda unit)=amount
of patient's plasma that
destroys half of factor VIII in
an equal mixture of normal
and patient's plasma
(1U×plasma volume×0.5)

plasma volume=40 ml/kg of
body weight

Eradication

Active Treatment

autoantibody   alloantibody
                      hemophilic
nonhemophilic

Immunosuppressive treatment:
(~60% response) prednisone
1 mg/kg/day

3 weeks

Inhibitor level — inhibitor disappears

decreased
to 50% or
less of
original
level

Taper off
prednisone

High dose IgG
0.4–1.0 g/kg
for 5 days in
slow infusion
(4–6 h)

inhibitor disappears

inhibitor persists

Cyclophosphamide 2 mg/kg/d
PO for 6 weeks (adjust dose
according to weekly CBC;
contraindicated in pregnancy)

inhibitor
persists

Immunotolerance Induction with Immunosuppressive
Treatment:

Try one of the following protocols (no established
recommendations exist):

Bonn protocol:
  100 U factor VIII/kg with 40–60 U FEIBA/kg q 12 h
  Check inhibitor on regular basis (usually peaks in
  1–2 months)
  When inhibitor level reaches 1 BU, switch to 150
  factor VIII/kg q d without FEIBA; when inhibitor
  cannot be detected continue low prophylactic
  dose several times a week for several weeks
  (usual treatment time: 7–24 months)

Immunosuppressive treatment with factor VIII:
  Prednisone + IV bolus of cyclophosphamide +
  daily factor VIII for 36 days to raise level between
  30–50 U/ml

US protocol:
  50 U/kg factor VIII q d for 4–6 months (anamnestic
  response expected in 1 month of treatment)

Go to
Fig.
44-1B

α-interferon 0.6 MU/m^2 SC every other day for 4
doses, and then 1.2 MU/m^2 for next 6 months

inhibitor persists

Try CVP (some authors advocate it as a first line treatment):
Factor VIII 50–100 U/kg followed by cyclophosphamide
500 mg on day 1 and 200 mg on days 2–5 IV; vincristine
2 mg on day 1 IV, and prednisone 100 mg/d PO on days
1–5

Repeat as necessary q 4 weeks (4–6 cycles)

A

Figs. 44-1A and B. Management of inhibitors against factor VIII. This algorithm is based upon combining the *physiological* and *cost/effectiveness approach*. The importance of the goal (eradication *vs* bleeding) and inhibitor level underline the physiologic approach. The choice of the mechanism to raise the factor VIII level (DDAVP, human factor VIII, porcine factor VIII) is based upon cost consideration as well. The risks associated with the use of factor IX complexes leave this option to those patients not

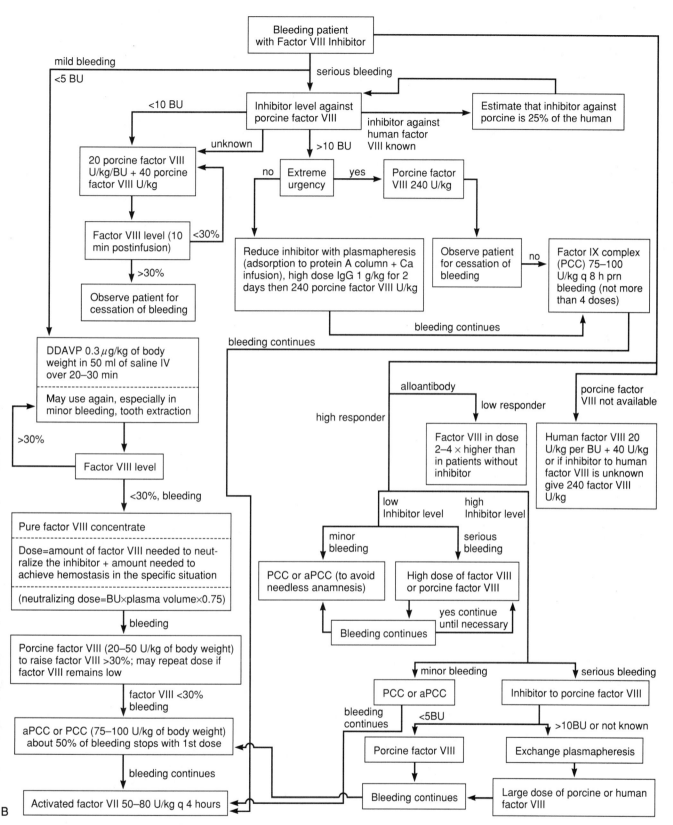

Bleeding patient
with Factor VIII Inhibitor

mild bleeding
<5 BU

serious bleeding

Inhibitor level against
porcine factor VIII

inhibitor against
human factor
VIII known

Estimate that inhibitor against
porcine is 25% of the human

<10 BU

>10 BU

unknown

20 porcine factor VIII
U/kg/BU + 40 porcine
factor VIII U/kg

no   Extreme
urgency   yes   Porcine factor
VIII 240 U/kg

Factor VIII level (10
min postinfusion)   <30%

>30%

Observe patient for
cessation of bleeding

Reduce inhibitor with plasmapheresis
(adsorption to protein A column + Ca
infusion), high dose IgG 1 g/kg for 2
days then 240 porcine factor VIII U/kg

Observe patient
for cessation of
bleeding   no   Factor IX complex
(PCC) 75–100
U/kg q 8 h prn
bleeding (not more
than 4 doses)

bleeding continues

bleeding continues

DDAVP 0.3 μg/kg of body
weight in 50 ml of saline IV
over 20–30 min

May use again, especially in
minor bleeding, tooth extraction

>30%

Factor VIII level

<30%, bleeding

Pure factor VIII concentrate

Dose=amount of factor VIII needed to neut-
ralize the inhibitor + amount needed to
achieve hemostasis in the specific situation

(neutralizing dose=BU×plasma volume×0.75)

bleeding

Porcine factor VIII (20–50 U/kg of body weight)
to raise factor VIII >30%; may repeat dose if
factor VIII remains low

factor VIII <30%
bleeding

aPCC or PCC (75–100 U/kg of body weight)
about 50% of bleeding stops with 1st dose

bleeding continues

Activated factor VII 50–80 U/kg q 4 hours

alloantibody

low responder

high responder

Factor VIII in dose
2–4 × higher than
in patients without
inhibitor

porcine factor
VIII not available

Human factor VIII 20
U/kg per BU + 40 U/kg
or if inhibitor to human
factor VIII is unknown
give 240 factor VIII
U/kg

low
Inhibitor level

high
Inhibitor level

minor
bleeding

serious
bleeding

PCC or aPCC (to avoid
needless anamnesis)

High dose of factor VIII
or porcine factor VIII

Bleeding continues

yes continue
until necessary

minor bleeding

serious bleeding

PCC or aPCC

Inhibitor to porcine factor VIII

bleeding
continues   <5BU   >10BU or not known

Porcine factor VIII

Exchange plasmapheresis

Bleeding continues   Large dose of porcine or human
factor VIII

B

adequately responding to factor VIII. Note that because of the low incidence of these conditions, no randomized trials have been published, and the proposed treatment is based upon anecdotal data and preliminary study report. (If not indicated otherwise, same doses of factors are used in acquired and congenital hemophilia. Since porcine factor VIII may cause anaphylactic reaction, never administer it without "antianaphylactic kit" at hand.) PCC, prothrombin complex concentrate (factor IX complex).

Suggested Readings

Brackman HH, Gormesn J: Massive factor VIII infusion in haemophiliac with factor VIII inhibitor, high responder. Lancet ii:933, 1977

Hay CRM, Bolton-Maggs P: Porcine factor VIII:C in the management of patients with factor VIII inhibitors. Trans Med Reviews V:145, 1991

Kasper CK: Treatment of factor VIII inhibitors. Prog Hemost Thromb 9:57, 1989

Kernoff PBA: Porcine factor VIII: preparation and use in treatment of inhibitor patients. Prog Clin Biol Res 150:207, 1984

Kessler CM (ed): Acquired factor VIII inhibitors in the nonhemophiliac: historical perspectives, current therapies and future approaches. Am J Med 91(5A):1s, 1991

Schwerdfeger R, Hintz S and Huhn D: Successful treatment of a patient with postpartum factor VIII inhibitor with recombinant human interferon 2α. Am J Hematol 37:190, 1991

45 | Disseminated Intravascular Coagulation (DIC)

Disseminated intravascular coagulation (DIC) is the second most common cause of acquired coagulation disorder after liver disease. It can be seen in almost every type of severe illness, from infectious diseases to metastatic cancer. The conditio sine qua non for DIC is the *simultaneous formation of thrombin and plasmin*. The main mechanisms initiating thrombin generation can be found within endothelial and tissue injury (Fig. 45-1). Thrombin converts fibrinogen to fibrin, activates factors V and VIII, activates factor XIII, and aggregates platelets. Secondary fibrinolysis invariably accompanies thrombin formation, with plasmin lysin factors V, VIII, IX, HK, fibrinogen, and fibrin. These actions of thrombin and plasmin form a *physiologic basis* for a diagnosis of DIC (Fig. 45-2). A clinical diagnosis will, however, involve a *probabilistic approach*, with adequate use of laboratory tests in the diagnosis of DIC (Table 45-1). If the index of suspicion for diagnosis is low, one should run highly sensitive tests to exclude DIC. (Historically, a protamine sulfate test to precipitate fibrin monomers is the test with the highest sensitivity, close to 100%. This test, however, is operator-dependent and time-consuming, and is going out of style). The classic definition of DIC (remember, DIC is a *laboratory* diagnosis) is the prolongation of PT or PTT, thrombocytopenia, and hypofibrinogenemia. If this is found, a diagnosis can be considered to be established. If only two tests are low, then highly specific, confirmatory tests, such as a test for cross-linked fibrin degradation—D-Dimer, should be determined (Fig. 45-2) (see also Chapter 1, Fig. 1-4). Table 45-2 shows a differential diagnosis of acute DIC, chronic DIC, and fibrinogenolysis, be-cause these conditions can show similar laboratory changes.

As far as the treatment of DIC is concerned, a general consensus has been reached that *treatment of the underlying condition* is the most important therapeutic measure. Ample use of supportive blood products (FFP, cryoprecipitate, platelets concentrates) is advocated by some authors, but cautioned by others (Fig. 45-3) (especially the use of products containing fibrinogen or other clotting factors). Our experience favors the former approach. The question still remains whether or not to use heparin routinely. There have been no randomized studies done on heparin therapy of DIC to justify its routine use. It seems, however, that there are some clear-cut indications for the institution of heparin. These would be cases with obvious clinical evidence of thrombosis, manifested as dermal necrosis, acral ischemia, purpura fulminans, retained dead fetus with low fibrinogen, acute promyelocytic leukemia, etc. (See Fig. 45-3).

Also, it has traditionally been considered contraindicated to administer antifibrinolytic therapy because of a fear of inducing massive generalized thrombosis, which could possibly happen if secondary fibrinolysis is blocked. Recently it became clear that, if the level of plasmin inhibitor is low, antifibrinolytic therapy can have a beneficial effect (see Fig. 45-3). Despite advances in treatment in recent years, the overall mortality rate in DIC is still high—between 25–75%, ranging from as low as 1% in cases of placental abruption to as high as 90% in case of septic shock.

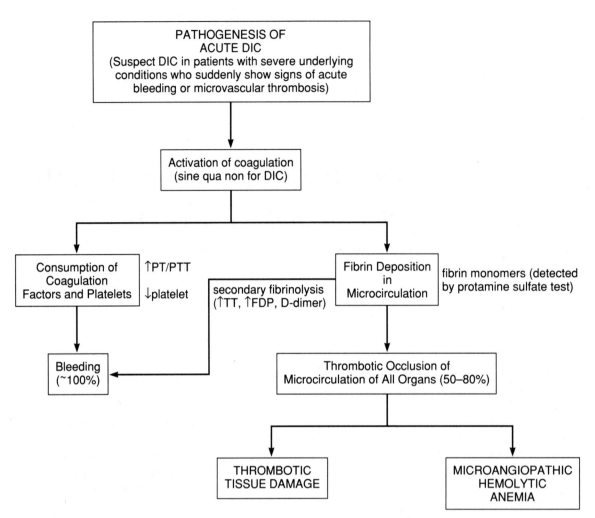

Fig. 45-1. Pathogenesis of disseminated intravascular coagulation (DIC). Simultaneous formation of thrombin and plasmin is the de facto definition of DIC. This formation is recognized by the panel of tests shown in Table 45-1.

Table 45-1. Operating Characteristics of Laboratory Tests Used in Diagnosis of Disseminated Intravascular Coagulation

Diagnostic Test	Sensitivity (%)	Specificity (%)	Comment
Platelet count	73–97	48	Thrombocytopenia, often first laboratory abnormality to be detected
Fibrinogen	22–79	87	If fall in level is taken into consideration, sensitivity is much higher; single value may thus not be helpful
Prothrombin time	76–90	~90	Exclude liver disease, vitamin K deficiency, coumadine treatment
aPTT	63–90	~90(?)	Exclude heparin treatment
Fibrin monomers (e.g., protamine sulfate)	>95	65	May be cumbersome to perform; proof of thrombin effect
FDP	95	56	Proof of plasmin effect
D-dimer	85–93	97	Proof of thrombin + plasmin effect
FDP + D-dimer	100	97	Confirms DIC

(Data from Semin Thromb Hemost 1988;14:299, Am J Med 1972;52:679, and Am J Clin Pathol 1989;91:280.)

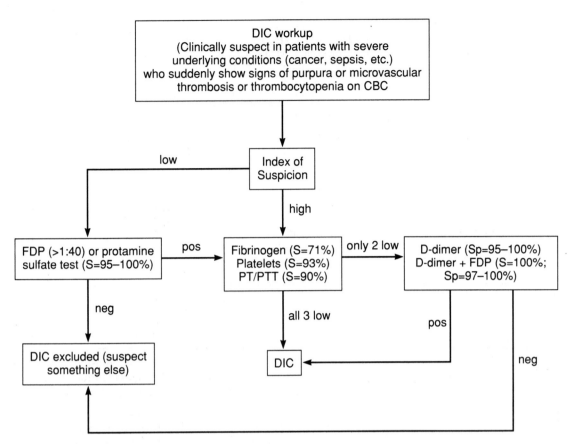

Fig. 45-2. Clinical diagnosis of DIC. *Probabilistic* approach, with the ordering of highly sensitive tests in a low probabilistic setting (*exclusion of diagnosis*) and highly specific tests in a high probabilistic setting (*confirmatory strategy*) is the most appropriate one. Readily available platelet counts in the routine CBC and hospital setting (e.g., ICU patient) also play a role in triggering DIC in initial diagnostic consideration. (See Chapter 1 for discussion of the principles of availability and representative heuristics.)

Table 45-2. Laboratory Profiles in Acute and Chronic DIC and Fibrinogenolysis

Diagnostic Test	Acute DIC	Chronic DIC	Fibrinogenolysis
Platelets	Low (moderate to severe)	Borderline low or normal	Normal
PT	Prolonged	Normal/short	Normal
PTT	Prolonged	Normal/short	Normal
TT	Prolonged	Normal/prolonged	Prolonged
Fibrinogen	Low	Low/normal/high	Low
Protamine sulfate test	Positive	Positive	Negative
Euglobin lysis time[a]	Normal	Normal	Short
FDP	Positive	Positive	Markedly positive
Schistocytes	Present (50%)	Present (90%)	Absent
Factor V	Low	Normal	Low
Factor VIII	Low	Normal	Low/normal
Fibrinopeptide A	Elevated	Elevated	Normal
Fibronopeptide B	Elevated	Elevated	Normal
B-β 1–42	Elevated	Elevated	Elevated

[a] Classic finding; test now considered outmoded.
(Data from Arch Intern Med 149:1724, 1989 and Semin Thromb Hemost 14:299, 1988.)

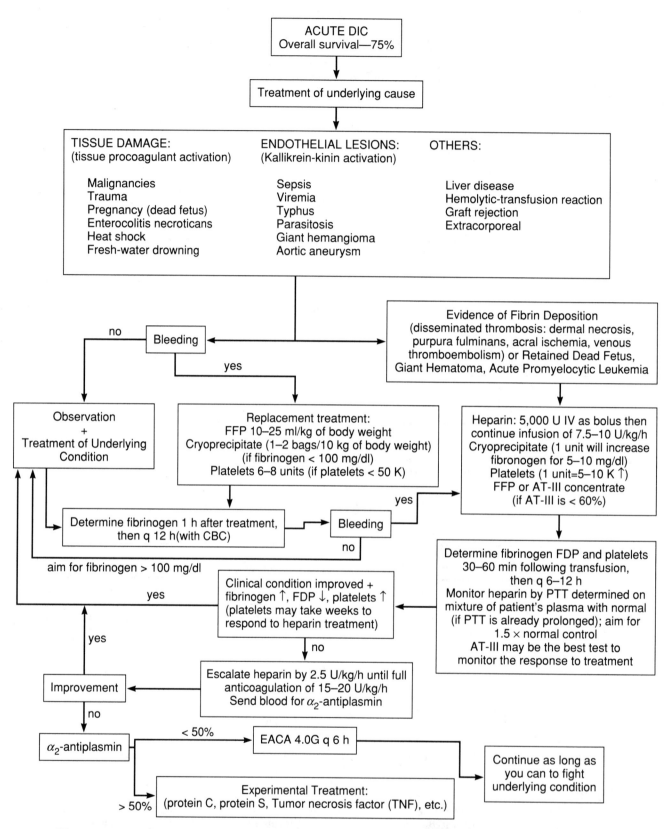

Fig. 45-3. Management of DIC. The *physiological* principle of "treatment of the underlying cause" is the mainstay of management. Other principles based upon current physiologic knowledge, such as the use of heparin and avoidance of plasma components, do not give uniformly good results. Their use is, therefore, highly individualized. Note that there is no need to treat laboratory data per se (without clinical complications). FFP, fresh frozen plasma; K, thousand/mm³.

Suggested Readings

Bick RL: Disseminated intravascular coagulation and related syndromes: a clinical review. Semin Thromb Hemost 14:299, 1988

Feinstein DI: Diagnosis and management of disseminated intravascular coagulation: the role of heparin therapy. Blood 60:284, 1982

Feinstein DI: Disseminated intravascular coagulation: how to intervene in a complex process. J Crit Illness 4:21, 1989

Wolf PL: The importance of alpha-antiplasmin in the defibrination syndrome. Arch Intern Med 149:1724, 1989

46 Thrombotic Thrombocytopenic Purpura

Thrombotic thrombocytopenic purpura (TTP) is a rare disorder with a prevalence of about 1 case per 5,000–50,000 hospital admissions. Its etiology and pathogenesis are both complex and poorly understood, but one hypothesis points to abnormal multimers of von Willebrand's disease, due to a lack of appropriate "depolymerase." A diagnosis is made upon the presence of a pentad of clinical signs: *Coombs negative microangiopathic hemolytic anemia* (96–98%) (evidence of *schistocytes* in the peripheral smear, is considered to be essential in the diagnosis of TTP (seen in −99% cases), *thrombocytopenia* (83–96%), *neurological symptoms* (52–92%), *renal impairment* (76–88%) and *fever* (59–98%). All five findings are present in 40–70% of patients. Depending on the distribution and severity of organ involvement, a patient can show few symptoms or be extremely sick. In the differential diagnosis, it is important to consider other causes of thrombocytopenia, such as ITP, DIC (patients with TTP have a normal fibrinogen and PT/PTT*), Evans syndrome (Coombs test is negative in TTP), hemolytic uremic syndrome (HUS) (considered to be a part of same disease spectrum, often called TTP/HUS syndrome), HELLP (hemolysis, elevated liver enzymes, low platelets) in pregnancy, and other causes of microangiopathic hemolytic anemia, such as malignant hypertension, vasculitis, connective tissue disorders, etc.

The cornerstone of treatment seems to be infusion of fresh-frozen plasma (FFP) at the quantity a patient can tolerate (usually one plasma volume per 24 hours). A recent prospective randomized trial showed that plasma exchange with fresh-frozen plasma is more effective than a plasma infusion alone. Some believe it is important that a plasma infusion is run between plasmapheresis sessions at whatever rate the patient can tolerate, to reduce a chance for relapse. A beneficial effect of FFP can be in providing lacking "depolymerase." The U.S. TTP Study Group recommends concomitant use of methylprednisone.

A variety of other measures (vincristine, antiplatelets agents, immunosuppressive, high-dose IgG, splenectomy, etc.) have been tried, but results are conflicting. About 15–20% of patients will experience chronic, relapsing courses, and they can be treated with FFP on outpatient basis with quantities varying from one to several units. With this approach, the mortality rate of TTP has dropped from 80–90% in the sixties to about 15–20% in the eighties.

---

* In one study, however, fibrinogen < 150 mg/ml was found in 7% of cases; in these cases, measurements of plasminogen activator or 6-keto-prostaglandin $F_{1\alpha}$, both decreased in TTP but normal/increased in DIC, are said to be of help.

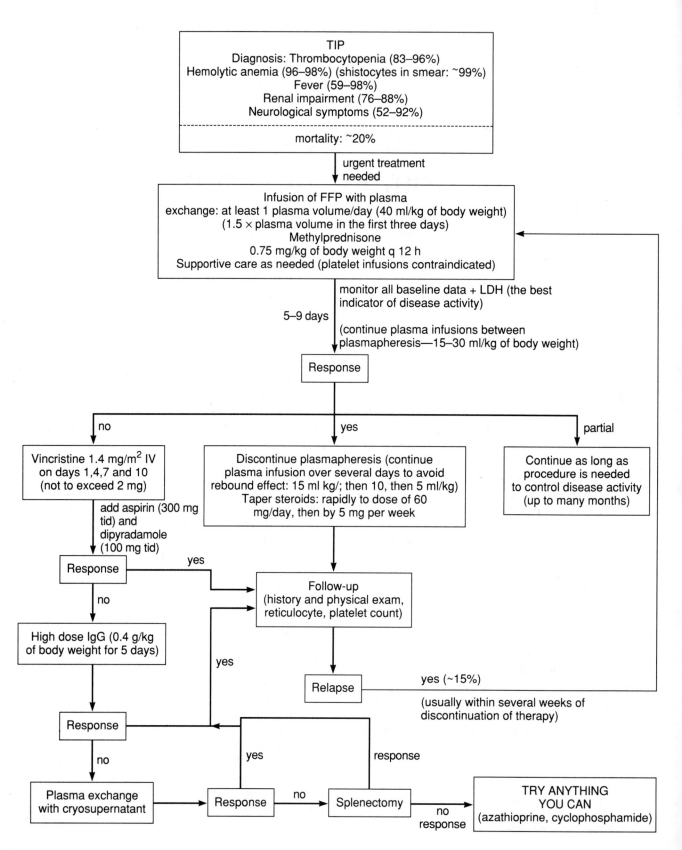

Fig. 46-1. The management of thrombotic thrombocytopenic purpura (TTP). The recommended strategy is based upon results of one randomized trial and uncontrolled accumulated experiences in the treatment of this rare disorder. *Probabilistic* and *risk/benefit estimates* dominate the approach in treatment. Diagnosis is made upon a well-developed *production rule* of identification of a pentad of symptoms.

Suggested Readings

Bell WR, Braine HG, Ness PM, et al.: Improved survival in thrombotic thrombocytopenic purpura-hemolytic uremic syndrome. Clinical experience in 108 patients. N Engl J Med 325:398, 1991

Case 36-1991 (Thrombotic thrombocytopenic purpura). N Engl J Med 325, 1991

Finn G, Wang JC, Hong KJ: High-dose intravenous gamma-immunoglobulin infusion in the treatment of thrombotic thrombocytopenic purpura. Arch Intern Med 147:2165, 1987

Lichtin AE, Schreiber A, Hurwitz S, et al.: Efficacy of intensive plasmapheresis in thrombotic thrombocytopenic purpura. Arch Intern Med 147:2122, 1987

Rock GA, Shumak KH, Buskard NA, et al.: Comparison of plasma exchange with plasma infusion in the treatment of thrombotic thrombocytopenic purpura. N Engl J Med 325:393, 1991

Rose M, Eldor A: High incidence of relapses in thrombotic thrombocytopenic purpura. Clinical study of 38 patients. Am J Med 83:437, 1987

47 | Thrombotic Disease

The consequences of *arterial* and *venous thrombosis* (myocardial infarction, stroke, pulmonary embolism) are by far leading causes of mortality and morbidity. Unfortunately, these events are usually diagnosed during the full-blown clinical picture of the underlying pathologic event. The key element in the clinical approach to these problems is searching for risk factors with the aim of reducing or eliminating them (e.g., weight control, quitting smoking, cholesterol modified diet, etc.). Family history is also very important; when risk factors are easy to identify, a special hematologic workup is rarely necessary. On the other hand, if risk factors are not present, and especially in the setting of thrombosis occurring in a young patient with a positive family history, the possibility of a primary hereditary hypercoagulable disorder should be strongly considered (Fig. 47-1). However, even with the best equipped laboratories, this will be successful in only about 15–25% of cases. Currently, no single screening test for the exclusion of hypercoagulable conditions, or one which points to further testing, can be recommended.

Deep venous thrombosis (DVT) account for more than 300,000 hospitalizations per year. The clinical diagnosis of DVT is notoriously imprecise (S = 14–78%, Sp = 4–21%). One cannot rely on the clinical finding; whenever DVT is suspected, objective testing is essential (Fig. 47-2). More than 90% of pulmonary emboli (PE) originate from lower-extremity sites. PE is responsible for more than 50,000 deaths in the U.S. annually, with an overall incidence of about 500,000 annually. Data indicates that only 10–30% of these cases are recognized antemortem. Therefore, early recognition and therapy of DVT (and PE) with anticoagulant treatment becomes crucial (see Figs. 47-2 and 47-3).

In recent years fibrinolytic therapy has gained popularity, particularly in the treatment of acute myocardial infarction. While the continuing debate regarding the best choice for fibrinolytic treatment is going on (t-PA *vs* streptokinase *vs* urokinase *vs* scu-PA), it should be noted that this therapy is not harmless, and physicians should become familiar not only with its administration but also be able to cope with its side effects (i.e., bleeding) (see Fig. 47-4).

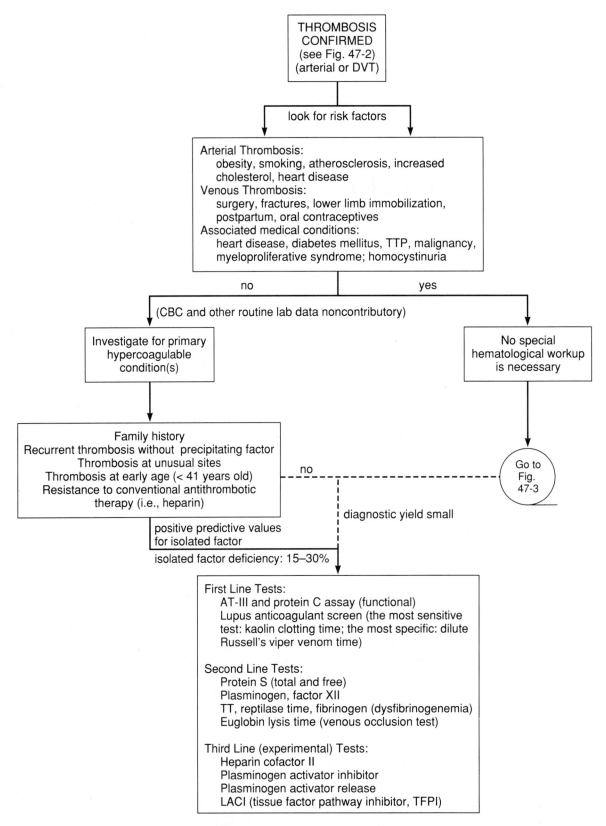

Fig. 47-1. Diagnosis of hypercoagulable disorders. Strategy is based upon consideration of the prevalence/incidence of the particular disorder and the validity of diagnostic tests employed in the diagnostic workup (*probabilistic strategy*).

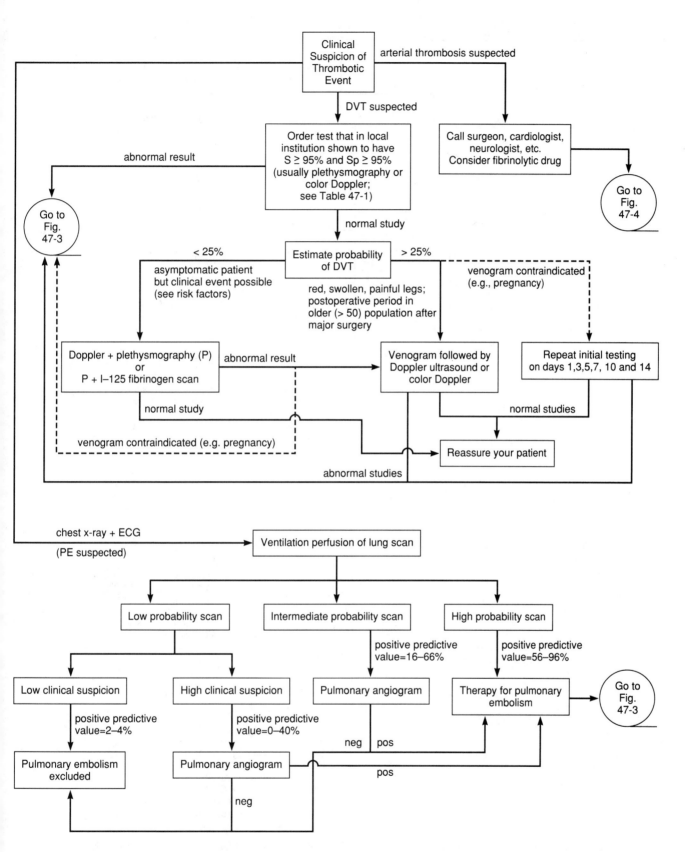

Fig. 47-2. Diagnosis of (DVT) and (PE). The proposed algorithm is based on the formal decision analysis of the value of diagnostic tests for DVT (see Venta et al.) and data from The Prospective Investigation of Pulmonary Embolism Diagnosis (PIOPED) (JAMA 263:2753, 1990). Note interlinking of the *probabilistic and threshold* reasoning concepts. (Broken arrows denote alternative strategy.)

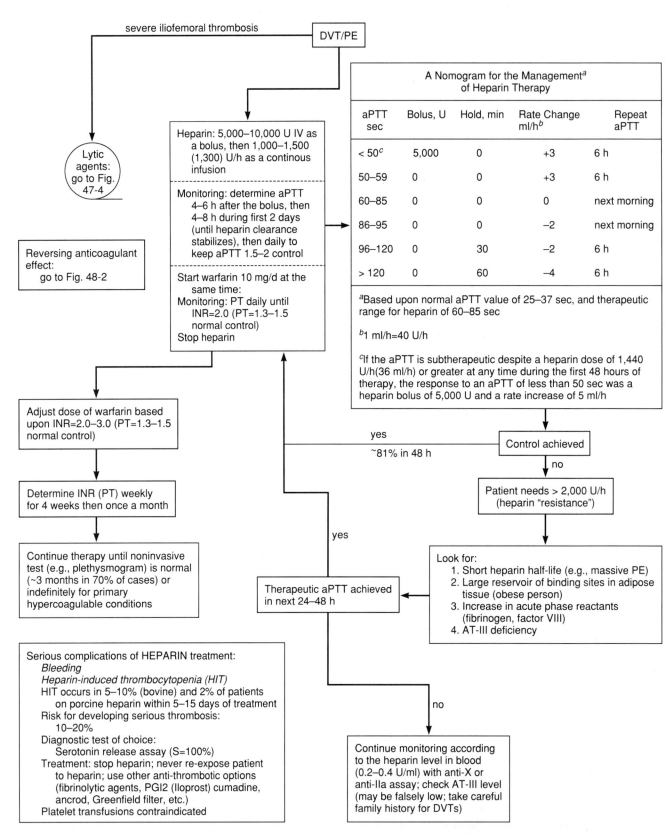

Fig. 47-3. Anticoagulant treatment of (DVT) and (PE). Monitoring of treatment is based upon the correlation of value monitoring tests (PTT, PT) with clinical parameters of interest (bleeding, clotting). Although the principles behind this reasoning are highly *physiologic,* actual decisions are based on *probabilistic* estimates (that patient will not clot/bleed) and *risk/benefit* estimates regarding anticoagulant therapy. (Nomogram taken from Cruickshank et al.: A standard heparin nomogram for the management of heparin therapy. Arch Intern Med 151:333, 1991, with permission.)

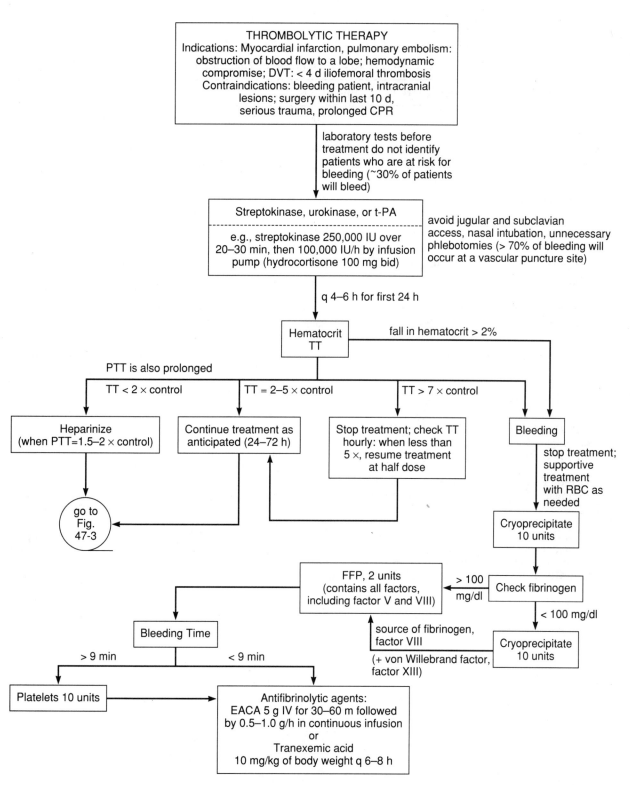

Fig. 47-4. Monitoring and management of bleeding during thrombolytic (T) therapy for DVT and PE (note that very few indications exist for administration of thrombolytics in this setting). Note also that the role of laboratory tests in monitoring and predicting bleeding during T treatment is very limited due to their poor operating characteristics (e.g., S = 61%, Sp = 45% for low fibrinogen; S = 8%, Sp = 98% for FDP > 400 μg/ml; S = 69%, Sp = 69% for bleeding time ≥ 9 min). Because of this, many physicians argue against use of any tests in the monitoring of T therapy. Presented is an algorithm based upon recommendations of Sane et al. (Ann Intern Med 111:1010, 1989) and Koch-Weser (N Engl J Med 304:1268, 1982), which are still used in many institutions.

Table 47-1. Operating Characteristics of Diagnostic Tests for Deep Venous Thrombosis

Diagnostic Test	Sensitivity (%)	Specificity (%)	Comment
Venography	100	100	Failure to visualize veins can occur in up to 9% of cases
Plethysmography (P)	71–98	77–98	Not sensitive for calf DVT
Doppler ultrasound (D)	76–93	83–91	Not sensitive for calf DVT
Duplex ultrasound	92–95	97–100	Not sensitive for calf DVT
I-125 fibrinogen scan (F)	70–97	44–85	Not suitable for study of the veins above mid-thigh or below midcalf
F + P	90–94	91–93	Relates to proximal and distal DVT
D + P	90	96	Proximal DVT
Color Doppler	90–100	91–100	Proximal DVT
Color Doppler	30–95	70–100	Calf DVT (depends on technical adequacy of study)

Compiled from BMJ 302:346, 1991; BMJ 301:1369, 1990; Radiology 174:433, 1990; Radiology 175:639, 1990; and Napodano RJ, 1991.

Suggested Readings

Hull RD, Raskob GE, Rosenbloom D, et al.: Heparin for 5 days as compared with 10 days in the initial treatment of proximal venous thrombosis. N Engl J Med 322:1260, 1990

Mannucci PM, Tripodi A: Laboratory screening of inherited thrombotic syndromes. Thromb Haemost 57:246, 1987

Napodano RJ: Deep venous thrombosis. In Panzer RJ, Black ER, Griner PF (eds.): Clinical diagnosis and laboratory: logical strategies for common medical problems. American College of Physicians, 1991

Sane DC, Califf RM, Topol EJ, et al.: Bleeding during thrombolytic therapy for acute myocardial infarction: mechanism and management. Ann Intern Med 111:1010, 1989

Schaffer AI: The hypercoagulable states. Ann Intern Med 102:814, 1985

Sidorov J: Streptokinase vs heparin for deep venous thrombosis. Can lytic therapy be justified? Arch Intern Med 149:1841, 1989

Venta LA, Venta ER, Mumfurd LM: Value of diagnostic tests for deep venous thrombosis: a decision analysis model. Radiology 174:433, 1990

Deficiency of Naturally Occurring Anticoagulants: Antithrombin III, Protein C, and Protein S

48

The estimated prevalence of *deficiencies of AT-III, protein S, and protein C* ranges between 1 in 2,000 to 1 in 20,000 individuals. The best estimate comes from studies on the prevalence of deficiencies of these proteins among patients with thrombosis. The prevalence of AT-III, protein C, and protein S deficiency was 6, 7, and 8.5%, respectively. In other words, in (young) individuals with proved venous thrombosis, there is about a 20% chance of deficiencies of one of these proteins. The risk for thrombosis increases with age, with a chance of more than 95% developing at least one thrombotic episode by the age of 60 in AT-III deficiency.

Deficiencies of all three proteins are usually inherited in the autosomal dominant fashion. Diagnosis is established by the level of these proteins in the plasma. The determination of their functional level is preferred to antigenic, although measurement of the free, functional form of protein S is cumbersome and immunological methods are currently used. In hereditary deficiency states, the levels usually fall in ranges between 40–65% normal, although most heterozygotes with levels above 50% in protein C deficiency do not develop thrombosis. One should be aware of acquired conditions that can cause deficiencies of these proteins (Fig. 48-1), but particularly important to remember is that pregnancy and birth control pills can decrease the level of both protein S and AT-III. A certain diagnosis of protein S deficiency in pregnancy is particularly difficult for this reason, as it is also in the diagnosis of AT-III deficiency during heparin use, where a marked decrease in AT-III can be expected.

Treatment of thrombosis in the setting of deficiencies of these proteins involves basically the same principles as the treatment of any other DVT (see Fig. 47-3). Recently AT-III concentrates became available, and we will probably see a wider use in the years to come. Protein C and protein S concentrates are expected to enter the clinical arena by the end of this century. It is important to remember *not* to start immediate treatment with oral anticoagulants in patients with protein C deficiency, since this can cause dangerous skin necrosis. Therefore, DVT in these patients should be treated with heparin first, together with simultaneous administration of FFP to provide an adequate source of protein C. Treatment of the *symptomatic* patient with deficiencies of AT-III, protein C, and protein S should be continued indefinitely (Fig. 48-2).

Whether an asymptomatic patient should be treated is still an unresolved issue. However, recent data from follow-up of one large family with AT-III deficiency indicated that lifelong anticoagulant treatment might not be necessary, with prophylaxis limited to high-risk periods for thrombosis.

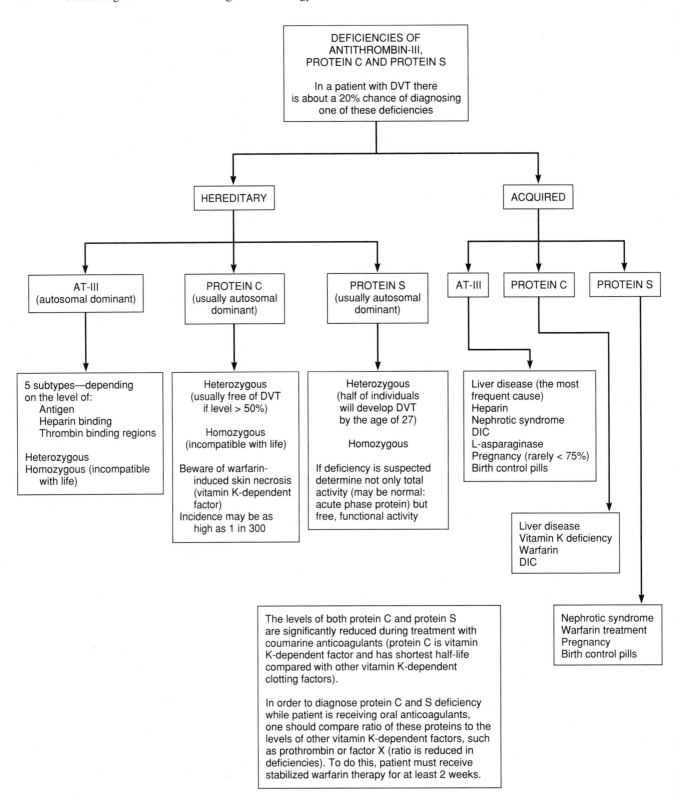

Fig. 48-1. Diagnosis of naturally occurring anticoagulant deficiencies. Although principles of diagnosis are largely *physiologic* (detection of deficient factor), their diagnostic predictive value is low because of the low prevalence of these conditions.

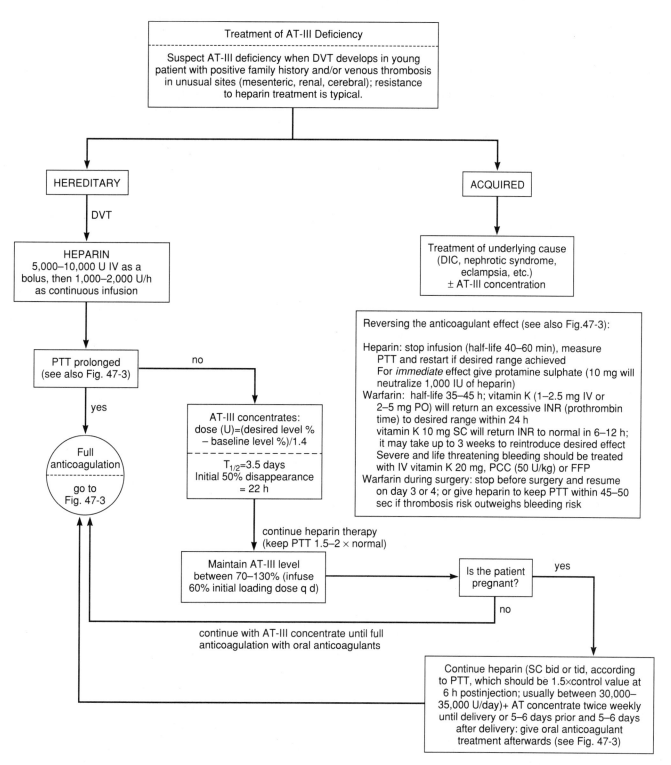

Fig. 48-2. Treatment of antithrombin III deficiency. Principles of treatment are *physiologic* in cases of replacement therapy with AT-III concentrate, but in cases of anticoagulants, therapy is based upon the estimate of the *probability of efficacy of anticoagulant treatment* (~80–90% for warfarin and heparin, respectively) and risk for severe bleeding (~5% for INR <3 for warfarin, and ~4% for heparin).

Suggested Readings

Clouse LH, Comp PC: The regulation of hemostasis: the protein C system. N Engl J Med 314:1298, 1986

Demers C, Ginsberg JS, Hirsh J et al: Thrombosis in antithrombin-III-deficient persons. Report of a large kindred and literature review. Ann Intern Med 116:754, 1992

Engesser L, Broekmans AW, et al.: Hereditary protein S deficiency: clinical manifestations. Ann Intern Med 106:677, 1987

Hirsh J, Piovella F: Congenital antithrombin-III deficiency. Incidence and clinical features. Am J Med 87(suppl.3B):34S, 1989

Menache D, O'Malley JP, Schorr JB, et al.: Evaluation of the safety, recovery, half-life, and clinical efficacy of antithrombin III (human) in patients with hereditary antithrombin III deficiency. Blood 75:33, 1990

Schwartz RS, Bauer KA, Rosenberg RD, et al.: Clinical experience with antithrombin III concentrate in treatment of congenital and acquired deficiency of antithrombin. Am J Med 37(suppl 3B):53S, 1989

49 Essential Thrombocythemia

Essential thrombocythemia (ET), or primary thrombocytosis, is a disease most commonly seen in people between 50–70 years of age, although a second affected population of predominantly young females appears to exist as well. The incidence of ET is estimated to be about 7 per million of population per year. With increased use of platelet determination in routine CBC, this incidence may increase soon. By definition, platelets exceed 600×10^9/L in all ET patients, but in more than 90% of patients this number will exceed 1 million/µl ($1,000 \times 10^9$/L). ET overlaps in clinical and laboratory features with other myeloproliferative disorders, therefore the major approach to diagnosis of ET is a negative one, that is, to *exclude* either another myeloproliferative disorder or reactive thrombocytosis (infections, inflammation, malignancy, blood loss, etc.) (see Fig. 21-8 for workup of myeloproliferative disorders and Table 49-1 for diagnostic criteria of ET).

The clinical presentation and course of disease varies; about two-thirds of all patients are completely asymptomatic and are diagnosed through routine CBC for unrelated reasons. Of symptomatic patients, about 30–50% will have hemorrhagic or vaso-occlusive symptoms. It seems that platelet count does not correlate with thrombohemorrhagic episodes—some patients will be asymptomatic even with platelet counts exceeding 5 million/µl. Nevertheless, there is evidence that thrombotic risk is lower when platelet counts are below 600×10^9/L ($<400 \times 10^9$/L according to some).

Since the course of disease is not predictable, *treatment* should be highly individualized. An unresolved issue is the treatment of asymptomatic, particularly young patients, because of the lack of data on the natural course of disease in this subset of patients. Since the major hematologic complication of ET is the development of myelofibrosis, which would be likely to shorten the life-span, some authors argue that *all patients* with ET should be treated. Others would reserve treatment for symptomatic patients, patients with counts greater than $1,000 \times 10^9$/L, or for elderly patients (thrombosis risk significantly increases after the age of 60). In the symptomatic group, it is important to determine whether an *acute*, major thrombohemorrhagic condition is developing or if the patient is experiencing *chronic* signs and symptoms of the disease (headache, paraesthesia, dizziness, pruritus, etc.). A splenectomy is considered an absolute contraindication to surgery. Figure 49-1 shows details of clinical management of patients with ET. One should also mention that the risk of hemorrhagic or vaso-occlusive complications in reactive thrombocytosis is substantially reduced and, accordingly, treatment would not be necessary outside of the treatment of an underlying cause. However, if the platelet count is greater than $2,000 \times 10^9$/L, treatment (along with reevaluation of the diagnosis) might be necessary.

The *prognosis* is considered excellent for young asymptomatic patients. More than 80% and 64% of patients will be alive at 5 and 10 years, respectively.

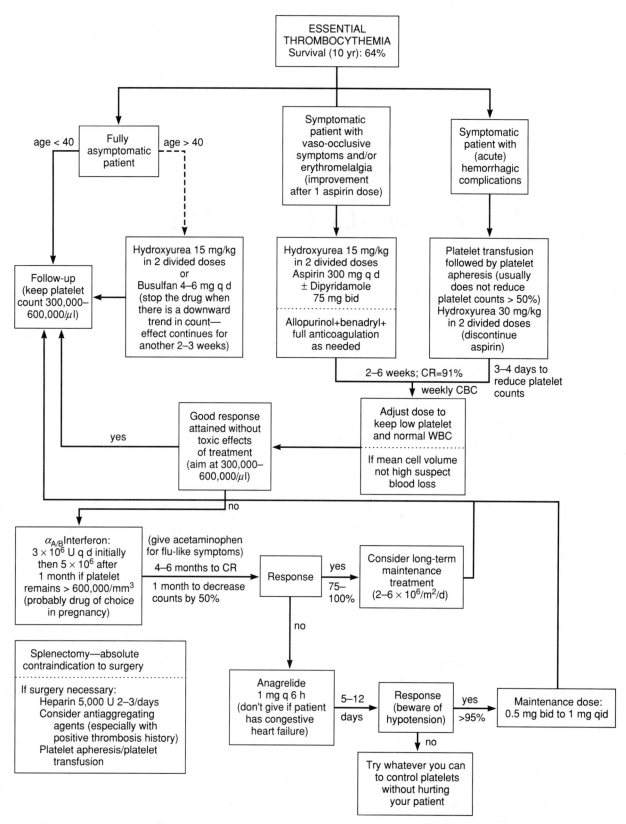

Fig. 49-1. The treatment of essential thrombocythemia. Construction of the algorithm is based upon the *risk/benefit estimate* of therapeutic options available in the disease, with a highly variable clinical course. Note that age and urgency of treatment are the two most important factors in a decision equation. A highly controversial issue is the treatment of patients older than 40–50 years who are fully asymptomatic (watchful waiting *vs* treatment). However, there is a consensus that the *threshold* for treatment should be low with even the most minor hemorrhagic or thrombotic complication. (Broken arrow denotes alternative strategy.)

Table 49-1. Production Rules For Diagnosis of Essential Thrombocythemia (ET)

I Negative Rule: Polycythemia Vera Study Group Production Rule For Diagnosis of ET
If the platelet count is $> 600 \times 10^9$/L *and* there is no evidence of raised RBC mass *and* there is no Philadelphia chromosome *and* there is no evidence of increased fibrosis in the marrow *and* there is no evidence for other diseases associated with reactive thrombocytosis, *then* consider ET established.

II Positive Rule: Scoring System for Diagnosis of ET*

Criteria	Score
Splenic enlargement on scan	2
Unstimulated BFU-E derived colonies present	2
Elevated ATP:ADP (>4 standard deviation from normal mean)	1
Elevated platelet distribution width	1
Clinical ischemia present	1

Scores $\geq =3$: Essential thrombocythemia (S = 89%, Sp = 100%)
Scores <3: Reactive thrombocytosis

* (Data from Dudley et al.: Br J Haematol 71:331, 1989.)

Suggested Readings

Buss DH, Stuart JJ, Lipscomb GE: The incidence of thrombotic and hemorrhagic disorders in association with extreme thrombocytosis: an analysis of 129 cases. Am J Hematol 20:365, 1985

Cortelazzo S, Viero P, Finazzi G, et al.: Incidence and risk factors for thrombotic complications in a historical cohort of 100 patients with essential thrombocythemia. J Clin Oncol 8:556, 1990

Mitus AS, Barbui T, Shulman LN, et al.: Hemostatic complications in young patients with essential thrombocythemia. Am J Med 88:371, 1990

Murphy S, Illand H, Rosenthal D, Laszlo J: Essential thrombocythemia: an interim report from the Polycythemia Vera Study Group. Semin Hematol 23:177, 1986

Pearson TC: Primary thrombocythemia: diagnosis and management. Br J Haematol 78:145, 1991

Silver RT: Interferon in the treatment of myeloproliferative diseases. Semin Hematol 27:6, 1990

Silverstein MN, Petitt RM, Solberg LA, et al.: Anagrelide: a new drug for treating thrombocytosis. N Engl J Med 318:1292, 1988

50 Red Blood Cells and Platelet Transfusion

The reasoning strategies employed in the administration of red blood cell (RBC) products and platelets involves an understanding of the physiologic need for these products (compromise in the oxygen-carrying capacity and hemostasis, respectively), an estimate of the risks associated with these products (probabilistic approach), and calculation of threshold levels of hemoglobin and platelets when transfusion is necessary. Since anemia and thrombocytopenia may have many different causes, an etiologic principle concerning correction of the underlying cause must be employed. Discussed below are situations when transfusion is used despite or concomitantly with underlying therapy.

Most *RBC transfusions* are given for blood loss during surgery, an acute gastrointestinal hemorrhage, chronic renal insufficiency, and complications of therapy in lymphoma or leukemia. Whole blood is used to treat acute blood loss of sufficient magnitude to cause hypovolemic shock (major surgery, trauma, gastrointestinal hemorrhage). Thirst, pallor, cool skin, tachycardia, and hypotension are indicators of massive blood loss. There is no clinical situation that absolutely requires the use of whole blood. In the treatment of acute, massive hemorrhage, whole blood can be replaced by packed red cells plus a crystalloid or colloid solution, supplemented as necessary by platelets and coagulation factor concentrates. It should be kept in mind that whole blood contains three times the sodium, four times the potassium, three times the ammonium, and three times the acid as packed red blood cells. Therefore, whole blood is contraindicated in patients with heart and renal failure and severe liver disease.

RBC are used for replacement of oxygen-carrying capacity in patients with anemia who are normovolemic. The use of RBC to raise the hematocrit to an arbitrary level is not a rational practice. The decision to transfuse is made on the basis of *all* relevant factors, such as the patient's age, cardiovascular status, the speed with which the anemia developed, the compensatory mechanisms of adaptation, the tolerance of anemia, and the patient's underlying disease. Rules (*thresholds*) that define indications for transfusion (Fig. 50-1) are the only general guidelines that are influenced by all the above-mentioned factors. Symptomatic anemic patients, particularly those with air hunger, angina, lightheadedness, or confusion, should be transfused. On the other hand, patients with good cardiac function may have adequate tissue oxygenation at hematocrit levels as low as 20–25%. Generally, sedentary patients will not manifest cardiovascular symptoms until the hemoglobin falls below 7 g/dl, but this is a highly individual variable.

Controversy exists over the most appropriate way to use *platelet transfusion*. The key issue in platelet transfusion therapy is whether platelets should be used *prophylactically* or reserved for episodes of clinical *bleeding*. There is a widespread practice of using platelet counts under $20 \times 10^9/L$ as a threshold for platelet transfusion, but recent evidence suggests that such an approach deserves critical evaluation. The members of the Consensus Development Panel of the U.S. National Institutes of Health in Bethesda believe that platelets are overused in some conditions. Concerning the available data, there is evidence suggesting that the majority of nonbleeding, clinically stable patients with chronic hypoprolifer-

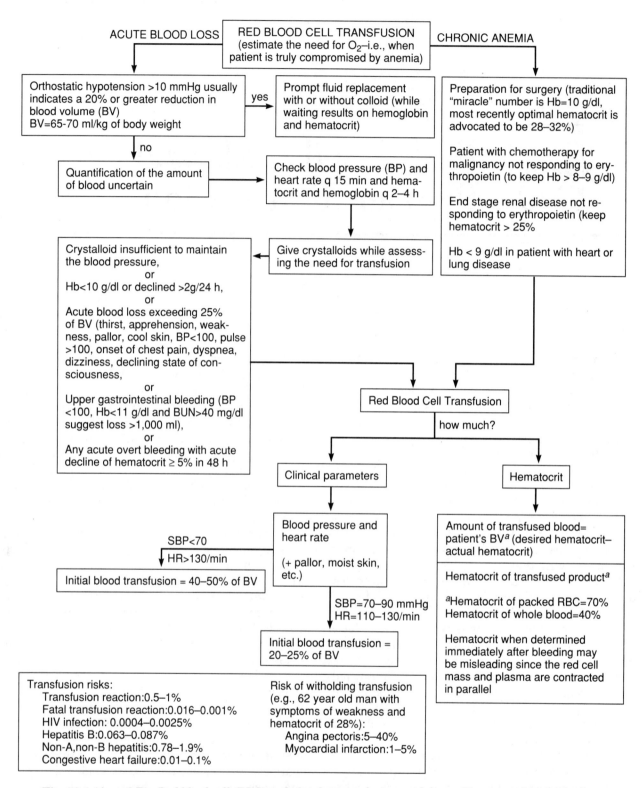

Fig. 50-1 (A and B). Red blood cell (RBC) and platelet transfusion guidelines. The reasoning strategies employed in the administration of RBC products and platelets involves an *understanding of the physiological need for these products* (compromise in the oxygen-carrying capacity and hemostasis, respectively), *estimate of the risk* associated with these products (probabilistic approach), and calculation of threshold levels of hemoglobin and platelets when transfusion is necessary. *Rules* (thresholds) that define indication for transfusion are only general guidelines that are influenced by all the factors depicted above and discussed in the text.

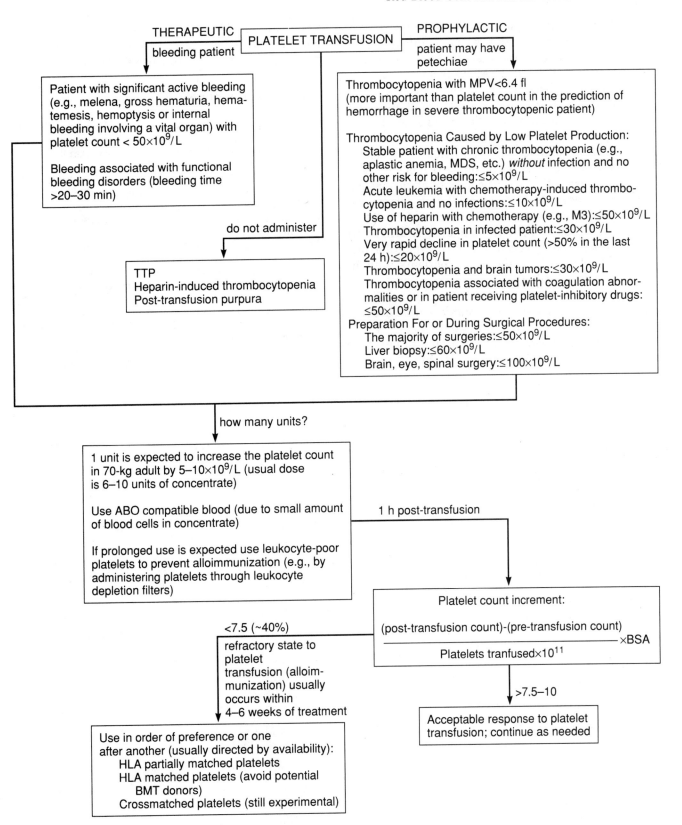

Fig. 50-1 (*Continued*)

ative thrombocytopenia (aplastic anemia, myelodysplastic syndrome) and without infection can maintain adequate hemostasis if the platelet level is greater than 5×10^9/L. Many factors may influence decisions about the need for platelet transfusion, such as patient's age, platelet trend, infection, bleeding time, location of hemorrhage, etiology of thrombocytopenia, mean platelet volume (MPV), coagulopathy, platelet function defect, and splenomegaly. Stool loss studies using Cr51 labeled erythrocytes indicate that a critical level of thrombocytopenia, under which substantial risk for spontaneous bleeding exists, is a value of 5×10^9/L (between $10–20 \times 10^9$/L in nonfebrile AML). Many authors point out this count as a threshold for prophylactic platelet transfusion in patients with no other risk for bleeding.

An unresolved issue is the prevention of alloimmunization against platelets. Many centers are routinely using leukocyte depletion filters, which, though rather expensive, are expected to benefit a maximum of about 10–15% of patients. Trials are underway to address the issue of whether the use of cheaper technology, such as UV-B irradiation, can provide the same or better benefit than filters.

Suggested Readings

Aderka D, Praff G, Santo M, et al.: Bleeding due to thrombocytopenia in acute leukemias and reevaluation of the prophylactic platelet transfusion policy. Am J Med Sci 291:147, 1986

Coffin C, Matz K, Rich E: Algorithm for evaluating the appropriateness of blood transfusion. Transfusion 29:298, 1989

Consensus Conference, Platelet transfusion therapy. JAMA 257:1777, 1987

Murphy S: Guidelines for platelet transfusion. JAMA 259:2453, 1988

Salem-Schatz SR, Avorn J, Soumerai SB: Influence of clinical knowledge, organizational context, and practice style on transfusion decision making. Implications for practice change strategies. JAMA 264:471, 1990

Schiffer CA: Prevention of alloimmunization against platelets. Blood 77:1, 1991

Silberstein LE, Kruskall MS, et al.: Strategies for the review of transfusion practices. JAMA 262:1993, 1989

51 Transfusion Reactions

It is estimated that more than a million red blood cell (RBC) transfusions are administered in the U.S. each year. It is, therefore, not surprising that *adverse reactions* are common companions to this highly prevalent practice. Adverse reactions may occur in up to 20% of all transfusions. Physiologically, these reactions can be thought of as *immunologic vs nonimmunologic*, but this is not very useful clinically, since symptoms of transfusion reaction are often nonspecific and may begin within minutes of transfusion, when there is not enough time to make a distinction between transfusion mechanisms by the use of complex laboratory procedures. An approach to this problem is then based on distinction between the most serious reaction *vs* the most probable reaction. In practice, this means a distinction between *acute immune hemolytic reaction vs febrile nonhemolytic reaction*.

The estimated risk for fatal hemolytic transfusion reaction is in a range from 1.6 in 10,000–1 in 100,000 transfusions, and 75% of transfusion-associated fatalities were due to administration of blood to the wrong patient (incidence of nonfatal ABO-incompatible transfusions is probably around 1/1,000–1/20,000). On the other hand, the estimated incidence for febrile nonhemolytic transfusion reaction is about 1% of all transfusions.

Fever is one of the most common signs in both conditions. In febrile nonhemolytic reactions, fever occurs toward the end of the transfusion and, characteristically, the temperature falls once the transfusion has stopped. However, due to the low specificity of this sign, the transfusion should be stopped and workup should be directed first at excluding the most serious condition ("diagnosis you can't afford to miss") (Fig. 51-1).

The two most essential tests for determining RBC destruction are the post-transfusion direct antiglobulin (Coombs) test and visual estimation of the plasma hemoglobin of the recipient, followed by its quantitation. When both are positive, the presence of immune hemolysis is highly likely. If these tests are negative, hemolytic reaction can be excluded with high certainty.

Fig. 50-1 shows an approach to the most important immunologic and nonimmunologic adverse reactions toward transfusion.

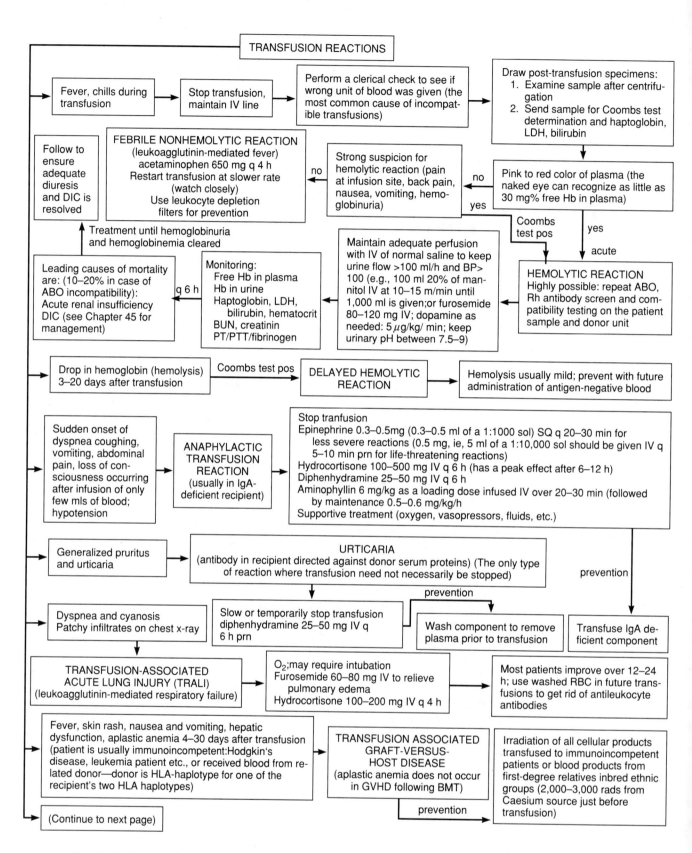

Fig. 51-1. Diagnostic and treatment approach to adverse transfusion reactions. These reactions can be immune- or nonimmune-mediated. Clinical reasoning strategy is based upon distinction of the most-serious reaction *vs* the most frequent (probable) reaction. In practice, this means distinction between *acute immune hemolytic reaction vs febrile nonhemolytic reaction.*

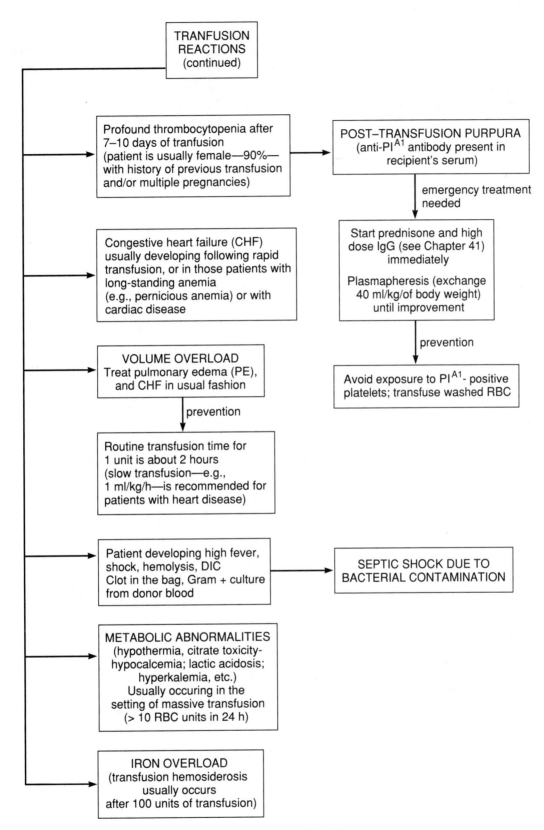

Fig. 51-1 (*Continued*).

Suggested Readings

Barbara JA, Contreras M: Infectious complications of blood transfusion: bacteria and parasites. Br Med J 300:386, 1990

Contreras M, Mollison PL: Immunologic complications of transfusion. Br Med J 300:173, 1990

Davies S, Brozovic M: Transfusion of red cells. Br Med J 300:248, 1990

Grindon AJ, Tomasulo PS, Bergin JJ, et al.: The hospital transfusion committee. Guidelines for improving practice. JAMA 253:540, 1985

Shulman IA: Adverse reactions to blood transfusion. Tex Med 85:35, 1989

Walker RH: Transfusion risks. Am J Clin Pathol 88:374, 1987

Index

Page numbers followed by f indicate figures; those followed by t indicate tables.

Test Sensitivity and Specificity Index

Page numbers followed by f indicate figures; those followed by t indicate tables.

Plethysmography, in deep venous thrombosis, 230t
Polycythemia rubra vera criteria, in polycythemia rubra vera, 83t
Protamine sulfate test, in disseminated intravascular coagulation, 216t
Prothrombin time (PT)
    in disseminated intravascular coagulation, 216t
    in factor VII deficiency, 193t
Prothrombin time (PT)/partial thromboplastin time (PTT), in bleeding disorders, 189f

Red blood cell folate, in folate acid deficiency, 28t
Red blood cell mass, in polycythemia rubra vera, 83t
Red blood cell porphobilinogen deaminase, in acute intermittent porphyria, 69t
Red blood cell protoporphyrin, in iron deficiency anemia, 22t
Red blood cells, in thalassemia, 37, 38f
Red (cell) distribution width (RDW)
    in iron deficiency anemia, 15t, 22t
    in vitamin B_{12} deficiency/folate acid deficiency, 28t
Reticulocyte count
    in hemolysis, 15t, 35t
    in hereditary spherocytosis, 47
Ristocetin cofactor assay, in von Willebrand's disease, 208t
Ristocetin-induced platelet aggregation (RIPA), in von Willebrand's disease, 208t

Schilling test (stage I and II), in pernicious anemia, 28t

Serotonin release assay, in heparin-induced thrombocytopenia, 228f
Serum erythropoietin
    in polycythemia rubra vera, 83t
    in secondary polycythemia, 83t
Serum ferritin
    in hereditary hemochromatosis, 61, 63f
    in iron deficiency anemia, 22t
Smoking, in smoker's polycythemia, 83t
Spherocytosis, in hereditary spherocytosis, 35t
Splenic percussion sign, in splenomegaly, 147t
Splenomegaly
    in chronic myelogenous leukemia, 113
    in hereditary spherocytosis, 15t, 35t, 47
    in idiopathic myelofibrosis/agnogenic myeloid metaplasia, 117
    in polycythemia rubra vera, 83t
Symptoms alone, in von Willebrand's disease, 208t

Thrombin time (TT)
    in low fibrinogen, 193t
    in postoperative bleeding, 193t
Total platelet IgG (TPIgG), in chronic idiopathic thrombocytopenic purpura, 195
Transferrin saturation
    in hereditary hemochromatosis, 61, 63f
    in iron deficiency anemia, 15t, 22t
Transferrin saturation plus ferritin, in hereditary hemochromatosis, 61, 63f
Traube's space percussion, in splenomegaly, 147t

$UB_{12}BC$, in polycythemia rubra vera, 83t
Ultrasound
    abdominal/pelvic, in relapse detection in nonHodgkin's lymphoma, 167t
    color Doppler, in deep venous thrombosis, 230t
    Doppler, in deep venous thrombosis, 230t
    Doppler plus plethysmography, in deep venous thrombosis, 230t
    Duplex, in deep venous thrombosis, 230t
    in extrahepatic obstruction, 77t
    in hepatoma, 64f
    in renal cyst, 83t
    transcranial Doppler, in stroke prediction, 44f
Urine, dark
    in acute intermittent porphyria, 69t
    in hereditary coproporphyria, 69t
    in variegate porphyria, 69t

Venography, in deep venous thrombosis, 230t
Vitamin B_{12}
    in polycythemia rubra vera, 83t
    in vitamin B_{12} deficiency, 15t, 28t
von Willebrand factor:antigen (vWF:Ag), in von Willebrand's disease, 208t
von Willebrand factor:ristocetin cofactor assay (vWF:RCoF), in von Willebrand's disease, 208t

Watson-Schwartz test, in acute intermittent porphyria, 69t
White blood cells, in polycythemia rubra vera, 83t